GW00600688

INTENSIVE CARE

APRIL 1980.
PAM SMITH.
A LEAVING GIFT FROM
THE KINGSLEY
CROWD.
(RINO'S)

Intensive Care

Edited by

G. GERSON M.B. D.(OBST.)R.C.O.G. F.F.A.R.C.S.

CONSULTANT ANAESTHETIST
ROYAL SUSSEX COUNTY HOSPITAL,
BRIGHTON

WILLIAM HEINEMANN MEDICAL BOOKS LTD
LONDON

First Published 1973
Reprinted 1975

© William Heinemann Medical Books Ltd 1973

ISBN 0 433 11610 2

Text set in 11/12 pt. IBM Baskerville, printed by photolithography,
and bound in Great Britain at The Pitman Press, Bath.

Contents

Preface

Many hospitals in this country have some form of intensive care unit, these units having been developed specifically for the treatment of critically ill patients who are suffering from disturbances of vital organ and system functions severe enough to endanger their lives. This has led to the concentration in these units of complex equipment and facilities for highly skilled multidisciplinary medical and nursing procedures.

The recently qualified doctor may find his first contacts with such a unit rather bewildering. With this consideration in mind, the authors felt that there was a real need to combine in one volume the different facets of management of the severely ill patient so as to provide a practical guide for junior hospital doctors. At the same time we trust that it will be of interest and value to medical students and nurses who are involved in the care of these patients.

The authors are all working or have worked in the intensive care unit at the Royal Sussex County Hospital, Brighton. They are all actively engaged in the everyday management of patients requiring intensive care and regard this as a task to be performed by a team of appropriate specialists.

The subjects covered are not intended to be exhaustive but are meant to form the basis of a reference for a general intensive care unit. The work of certain specialised units such as cardio-thoracic, paediatric and burns has not been specifically covered except in so far as the principles of treatment of severe physiological derangement remain the same regardless of the aetiological factors involved.

April 1973   G. G.

List of Contributors

Hedley BERRY, M. B., F.R.C.S.,
Consultant Surgeon,
Kings College Hospital, London.

Douglas CHAMBERLAIN, M.A., M.D., M.R.C.P.,
Consultant Cardiologist,
Royal Sussex County Hospital, Brighton.

Honorary Consultant Cardiologist,
Kings College Hospital, London.

Bernard CRYMBLE, M.B., F.R.C.S.,
Consultant Neurosurgeon,
Royal Sussex County Hospital, Brighton.

Gary GERSON, M.B., F.F.A.R.C.S.,
Consultant Anaesthetist,
Royal Sussex County Hospital, Brighton.

Philip MARSDEN, B.Sc., M.B., M.R.C.P.,
Lecturer in Medicine,
Kings College Hospital Medical School, London.

Iain M. MURRAY-LYON, B.Sc., M.B., M.R.C.P. (Lond.),
   M.R.C.P. (Edin.)
Honorary Senior Lecturer in Medicine,
Kings College Hospital, London.

Paul SHARPSTONE, M.B., M.R.C.P.,
Consultant Physician,
Royal Sussex County Hospital, Brighton.

Joanna SHELDON, M.D., M.R.C.P.,
Consultant Physician,
Royal Sussex County Hospital, Brighton.

Chapter 1

Acute Coronary Care

DOUGLAS CHAMBERLAIN

INTRODUCTION

MYOCARDIAL INFARCTION: A MEDICAL EMERGENCY

Indications for Admission to Hospital

Referral Procedures

The Use of Coronary Ambulances

THE ROLE OF A CORONARY CARE UNIT

The Functions and Organization of Coronary Care Units

Transfer to a General Medical Ward

THE TREATMENT OF PATIENTS WITH MYOCARDIAL INFARCTION

In Casualty

In the Coronary Care Unit

Routine Drugs after Myocardial Infarction

DISORDERS OF CARDIAC RHYTHM COMPLICATING MYOCARDIAL INFARCTION

Sinus Bradycardia

Supraventricular Extrasystoles

INTRODUCTION

The incidence of acute myocardial infarction is increasing rapidly, especially in young and middle-aged men. The mortality rate is more than 40 per cent, and three out of five of those who die do so within one hour. The majority of early deaths result from ventricular fibrillation, yet this is frequently a potentially reversible complication. These stark statements illustrate the challenge and the dilemma of coronary artery disease.

The dilemma concerns the timing of the fatalities. For lethal arrhythmias which occur without warning or within minutes of the first symptoms are hardly amenable to treatment. It follows that a major decrease in mortality rate from coronary artery disease must await new knowledge of its epidemiology and the development of effective prophylaxis. Any reduction which *can* be achieved at the present time depends to a large degree on effective therapy being made available to patients while they are still in the period of relatively high risk. The first part of this account will deal with this crucial problem, for it has received much less attention than it deserves. The treatment of the patient in hospital including the prevention and management of the complications of infarction will also be considered in detail.

MYOCARDIAL INFARCTION: A MEDICAL EMERGENCY

Most deaths from myocardial infarction occur swiftly after the onset of symptoms. All too frequently, victims of the disease never seek medical help, for patients are not accustomed to calling a doctor within minutes of the development of even severe symptoms, and ventricular fibrillation strikes with catastrophic suddenness. In a recent study reported from Doncaster, the greatest delay between the onset of symptoms and admission to hospital was due to the patients themselves, for half of them waited more than 1 hour 50 minutes before requesting medical assistance; by this time 75 per cent of all deaths would have occurred (Fig. 1.1). The median delay for the general practitioner responding to the call was 33 minutes, and for transfer to hospital a further 25 minutes. These figures compare favourably with studies elsewhere in Britain, but serve to highlight the almost intractable problem of providing skilled resuscitation at a time when it can be of most value.

Although the problem cannot be resolved satisfactorily, improvements can be made in reducing delay between the onset of symptoms and the provision of intensive care facilities. These improvements necessitate the abandoning of some entrenched attitudes on the indications for hospital admission, and also on the procedures for arranging and implementing admission. We believe that the acceptance of new concepts by hospital and general practitioners, and the provision of suitable facilities by

3

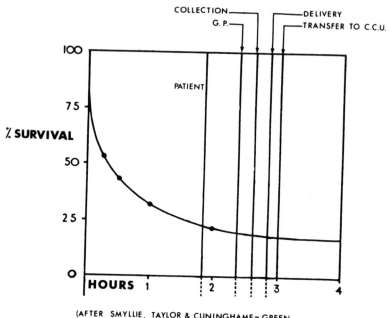

Fig. 1.1. A graph of percent survival plotted against time for patients in Doncaster who suffered fatal myocardial infarctions (coroner's cases, reported from within and from outside hospital). Superimposed on the graph are the median times for the factors which caused delay in patients admitted to hospital with myocardial infarction over the same 12-month period. Reproduced with permission of the authors and of the Editor of the *British Medical Journal*.

those who administer our hospitals and public health authorities can save at least a proportion of those who would otherwise die of coronary disease. These concepts can conveniently be discussed under three headings: the indication for admission to hospital, referral procedures, and the use of specially equipped coronary ambulances for moving patients to hospital.

Indications for Admission to Hospital

If coronary care facilities are to make any impact on mortality within the community, the emphasis must be placed on the admission to hospital of those who are likely to develop serious arrhythmias, principally patients who have suffered an infarct minutes, or at most a few hours, previously. In practice we recommend that a patient who has had symptoms for less than six hours which *may* be due to myocardial infaction should be moved to hospital unless some special reason exists for his being cared for at home (and age must be an important consideration). The sooner after the event the situation is recognized, the greater the urgency, and delay to await confirmation of the diagnosis is inappropriate. It should therefore be accepted that patients can be referred after a 'telephone' diagnosis by the family doctor without his delaying to make a visit, especially to patients who have previously experienced cardiac pain. On the other hand, if myocardial infarction is diagnosed more than six hours after the event, the patient has already crossed the major arrhythmic hurdles. If no complications are evident and he can be maintained and treated comfortably in his own home, it may be preferable to leave him there.

Mention must also be made of admission to hospital before infarction has occurred. An *abrupt* onset of angina pectoris is due to a coronary occlusion which has not caused muscle necrosis but has impaired the myocardial circulation to the point where metabolic demands cannot be met during exercise. The occlusion is usually thrombotic, or due to a minor subintimal haemorrhage in the wall of a coronary vessel. In either event, the pathological process may extend. For this reason patients who present with frank infarction often give a history of crescendo angina or coronary insufficiency (brief episodes of rest pain) during the days preceding the attack. It is therefore a reasonable precaution to admit patients to hospital if they have developed severe angina of effort within the previous few days, and particularly if they have also had pain at rest. The physician must be prepared to admit a patient on the basis of the history alone, for the majority of those who first present with cardiac pain have normal electrocardiograms. An electrocardiogram cannot detect a coronary occlusion *per se*; it can only indicate infarction, or myocardial ischaemia which is present at the time the tracing is taken.

In summary, if a logical admissions policy is to be pursued, the following groups of patients should receive priority for admission to hospital for coronary care:

   i. those who have had a myocardial infarction less than six hours previously;

  ii. those with arrhythmias, shock, or other major complications;

 iii. those whose home circumstances are unsuitable for nursing care;

 iv. those who can be considered likely candidates for a major infarction within a number of days, i.e. patients with increasing coronary insufficiency or crescendo angina.

Referral Procedures

In order to speed the admission to hospital of patients who have had a myocardial infarction, the administrative procedures must be simple, efficient, and rapid.

In circumstances which are now all too common, a busy general practitioner seeking to admit a patient may be frustrated first by long delays at an overloaded hospital switchboard, then by difficulties in locating the appropriate house officer, and finally be defeated by a shortage of hospital beds. For these reasons most admissions are now arranged by an emergency bed service. Such arrangements are not appropriate for the urgent admission of a patient with a very recent coronary occlusion.

With an ideal admission scheme, the practitioner should contact the ambulance service, and further arrangements for the patient's reception can be made while the ambulance itself is in transit. Ambulance control should inform the receiving house officer in the casualty department or Coronary Unit that a patient is on his way, and the general practitioner will, if circumstances permit, contact the hospital to give further details of the patient and his condition. In practice, an 'open-house' arrangement of this type may not be feasible for all patients because of the shortage of hospital facilities. Some type of 'rationing' of such a streamlined service may then be a necessity: for instance, patients under the age of 55 may be admitted under an 'open-house' policy, and the usual referral arrangement retained for older patients. Any suggestion of rationing of hospital services is abhorrent to many, but if the challenge of coronary disease is to be faced, a start must be made in introducing an admission procedure which pays due regard to the natural history of the disease. To refuse to implement an improved scheme because it is not immediately available to all would be to adopt a policy of complacency and despair.

The Use of Coronary Ambulances

Ventricular fibrillation is a common and lethal complication of myocardial infarction which can be treated in hospital but not at home. For this reason as many patients as possible should be moved to hospital while they are still in the period of high-risk for arrhythmias. However, it cannot be denied that movement of a patient increases the immediate risk. Some patients develop ventricular fibrillation in transit, and the proportion who do so will increase as the median delay shortens between the onset of symptoms and movement to hospital. The advantages of providing intensive care facilities during the journey are therefore obvious.

The first Coronary Ambulance in the United Kingdom was introduced in Belfast in 1966 by Professor J. F. Pantridge and his colleagues. The results have been impressive, but the benefits which can accrue from mobile coronary care of this type are difficult to measure and many critics doubt its value. The number of patients who are successfully defibrillated in the ambulance and in hospital does not provide a true measure of success. The proponents of the scheme point out that the treatment of dangerous bradycardia and ventricular arrhythmias prevents many cases of ventricular fibrillation which would otherwise occur. Its opponents argue that the ambulances treat problems of their own creation, for patients left in the quiet of their own homes are less likely to suffer rhythm disturbances than those who are moved into a strange and frightening environment. Unfortunately, we have no reliable statistics to compare home care and hospital care of myocardial infarction which take due account of the critical early few hours after the onset of symptoms. However, a comparison of mortality statistics from Belfast with the expected mortality derived from community studies strongly suggests that an integrated service with Coronary Ambulances and an efficient Coronary Care Unit can make a major contribution to the survival rate of patients with acute infarction.

The prevention and treatment of arrhythmias during transit to hospital is not the only benefit which can accrue from the use of a Coronary Ambulance. Another important advantage lies in the new sense of urgency which is gradually created in the community as a result of the existence of the ambulance and the publicity it inevitably receives. In Belfast, over the four-year period from 1966 to 1969, the proportion of patients who were treated within one hour of the onset of symptoms increased from 13 per cent to over 27 per cent. The median delay before patients came under intensive care has now been reduced to 1 hour 40 minutes.

The existence of a Coronary Ambulance system may also permit an extension of the 'rapid referral' policy outlined above. Appropriate patients, such as those with recent onset of angina of effort, could well be told by their general practitioners that they should contact the Coronary ambulance direct if they have cardiac pain at rest which lasts for more than 10 minutes and which does not respond to glyceryl trinitrate. This policy would almost eliminate the delay in bringing treatment to the patient at risk, but unfortunately not all patients have premonitory symptoms which have been recognized, and not all could be given this advice without engendering undue anxiety.

One serious criticism of mobile coronary care relates to the cost. The expense of a conventional Coronary Ambulance amounts to many thousands of pounds per annum, and any attempt to make this service available on a wide scale would make great demands in money and in medical manpower. A reasonable compromise may be to train ambulance personnel to monitor patients and to treat ventricular fibrillation and possibly other serious arrhythmias; experiments carried out in Dublin and in Brighton suggest that this offers an entirely feasible solution to the problems outlined above, although it remains to be seen how far these services can compare with some of the excellent Coronary Ambulances which are supported by trained medical staff.

THE ROLE OF A CORONARY CARE UNIT

In recent years, there has been an increasing tendency for major hospitals to have Coronary Care Units, and to admit patients with recent cardiac pain to these areas for a few days. Such units

8

are expensive to equip and to maintain, but unless they are used for patients who have — or are likely to develop — complications, their value is limited. It is common experience that only a minority of patients develop serious arrhythmias within a Coronary Care Unit. This may result from effective prophylaxis; too often it reflects undue delay between infarction and admission so that most potentially lethal arrhythmias occur outside hospital. A measure of this interval provides the most important single index of the efficiency of a coronary service, and the significance of mortality statistics cannot be assessed without it; yet frequently it is disregarded.

The Functions and Organization of a Coronary Care Unit

The principal functions of a coronary care unit are:

i. to provide constant ECG monitoring for the early detection and treatment of important arrhythmias;
ii. to provide facilities for the most effective treatment of other major complications of myocardial infarction, such as heart block, left ventricular failure, and cardiogenic shock;
iii. to provide training in the care of coronary patients and the principle of cardiac resuscitation for both medical and nursing staff.

The patient's comfort is of paramount importance and everything possible should be done to allay anxiety. This is no idle platitude, for fear can be an important factor in the genesis of ventricular arrhythmias. A terrified patient surrounded by intimidating gadgetry and receiving an infusion of an anti-arrhythmic drug is not entirely a figment of the imagination of the opponents of Coronary Care Units! Having conscious patients with recent cardiac pain in a general intensive care area is to be condemned, though for economy of skilled nursing and of specialized equipment it is convenient to have intensive care and coronary care areas adjoining, perhaps with a single nursing station between them. The patients should be in separate reasonably sound-proof cubicles so that they can be unaware of problems in adjoining beds, but each patient should be clearly

9

visible from the nursing station. If arrhythmia alarms are considered necessary, the system should not readily be triggered by artefact from patient movement.

A central console should show the ECGs of all patients, and facilities should be available for recording onto paper a rhythm strip from any individual at any time. A 'memory loop' on magnetic tape is an advantage so that the events of the previous minute or two can be recalled for detailed analysis. The bedside monitor should not have an audible R-wave bleep if the patient is conscious. Many people dislike the cables which attach them to the bedside unit. Miniaturized transmitters offer a feasible alternative and can provide unobtrusive monitoring. Such devices, capable of withstanding defibrillation shocks, are being developed, and will no doubt be used increasingly.

Coronary care nurses should be trained to recognize all common arrhythmias, and should be capable of defibrillating patients when necessary. They should also be permitted to give emergency drugs, such as atropine, lignocaine, and sodium bicarbonate, when the occasion demands, perhaps under the cover of 'p.r.n.' boardings, though in some centres the nursing administration does not encourage this practice. It is an unfortunate situation when skilled personnel have to waste vital minutes waiting for a physician while an easily remediable situation evolves into a potentially lethal rhythm disturbance.

Transfer to a General Medical Ward

The duration of hospital admission following myocardial infarction should probably be a minimum of 8 days, and longer if the course has been complicated by rhythm disturbances, failure, or persistent tachycardia. Patients with coronary insufficiency without infarction may continue in an unstable phase with recurrent ischaemic pain, and these, too, require a longer stay in hospital. The principal reason for keeping patients in hospital after the initial phase of their illness is that a small percentage will develop ventricular fibrillation unexpectedly a week or more after admission. It is impractical to have Coronary Care Units large enough to retain patients for the whole of this period; transfer to a general medical ward after about 48 hours free of major complications is, therefore, usual.

Constant ECG monitoring cannot be provided under these circumstances, but every medical ward with coronary patients should have a defibrillator and facilities for rapid emergency monitoring close at hand. Senior nursing staff on these wards should preferably undergo training within the coronary unit so that they, too, can defibrillate patients when necessary.

THE TREATMENT OF PATIENTS WITH MYOCARDIAL INFARCTION

In Casualty

In most hospitals, the patient is taken first to the casualty area. Ideally, ambulance control will have alerted the admitting house physician who will be awaiting his arrival, but otherwise the first duties will fall to one of the casualty staff. Whatever arrangements are made, patients with recent coronary occlusion must be afforded immediate priority and not left in casualty without a medical attendant. A very brief preliminary history will confirm that the patient has had or *may have had* cardiac pain: a high degree of suspicion is sufficient indication for admission to the coronary area. Feeling the patient's pulse is an adequate examination at this stage. Delay in the casualty department may be necessary for two reasons: the relief of pain by an analgesic (see below), or the emergency treatment of a serious rhythm disturbance. An oscilloscope must be available to monitor the heart rhythm during this critical period. The patient should be moved to the coronary unit as soon as his condition is sufficiently stable. Movement in the hospital should be at a gentle pace unless some complication supervenes, both to avoid anxiety and to avoid exacerbating the tendency to vomiting in a patient who has received analgesia with opiates.

In the Coronary Care Unit

The patient should be propped in bed in a position of maximum comfort. Nothing is gained by keeping him flat unless he is shocked, with a low venous pressure (a rare circumstance after myocardial infarction). The tendency for nurses to tilt the foot of the bed up if the patient is hypotensive must be firmly resisted! Once the patient is in the bed he is attached to the

11

monitoring facility; reassurance and explanation are important
at this stage: fear of gadgets, cables, and electrodes is understandable and widespread. An intravenous line should be
secured, and either left sealed or kept patent with a slow drip of
5% dextrose. In the presence of complications, such as shock,
serious arrhythmias, or conduction defects, the intravenous line
should comprise a long catheter (such as an Intracath or E–Z
cath) which can be introduced via a medial antecubital vein and
advanced about 18 inches so that its tip lies in the superior vena
cava. This permits not only the use of intravenous fluid and
drugs, but also the measurement of central venous pressure, the
taking of central venous blood smaples to follow trends in oxygen
saturation, and also the introduction of fine electrodes for intra-
atrial electrograms and emergency pacing. A portable X-ray
should be arranged (and taken whenever possible with the
patient sitting upright, not supine) so that the lung fields can be
assessed. When a long intravenous catheter has been used, the
X-ray will also show the site of the tip; if it lies outside the
thorax it should be repositioned. Once the heart rhythm is being
monitored and a venous line is in position, a full history can be
taken and an adequate examination carried out.

The patient should be allowed to rest as much as possible,
but for the first six hours after admission the pulse rate should
be taken – unobtrusively if possible – fairly frequently (perhaps
every 30 minutes) and the blood pressure recorded every two
hours. Observations may be needed more frequently in the
presence of complications. Throughout the patient's stay in the
Coronary Care Unit, the heart rhythm is observed carefully, and
noted at least hourly. The patient should be kept in bed (except
for commode) for the first 4 to 6 days; if the course is uncomplicated he is then gradually mobilized and discharged 8 to 14 days
after admission. If anti-coagulants are not given, the patient
should be mobilized gently from the fourth day. Elderly
patients are best allowed out of bed as soon as they are free of
pain and major complications.

Routine Drugs after Myocardial Infarction

1. *Sedative*. Diazepam (Valium) is the most useful drug for this
purpose and also serves to allay anxiety.

Dose: 2 to 5 mg t.i.d., by mouth.

2. *Analgesic.* Diamorphine is most suitable, and is slightly less prone to cause nausea and vomiting than morphine. It must be freshly diluted in its ampoule from a freeze-dried pellet because it hydrolyses rapidly in solution.

Dose: 5 mg by *slow* intravenous injection, followed by a further 2·5 mg after 10 minutes if severe pain persists.

If analgesics are given intramuscularly, pain relief may be very slow and shock may be unnecessarily prolonged. Furthermore, the physician may be uncertain whether to repeat an intramuscular dose and risk subsequent respiratory depression. Therapeutic effects can be titrated with precision if doses are given intravenously. However, injection must not be rapid because opiates both increase vagal tone and also release catecholamines from the adrenal medulla; if given in a bolus they may predispose to serious arrhythmias.

3. *Diuretic.* Even in uncomplicated cases of myocardial infarction some pulmonary congestion occurs in the acute stage. It may be a reasonable precaution to give a thiazide diuretic (e.g. Tabs Navidrex K 2 daily) as a routine measure for the first week.

4. *Anticoagulant.* The value of anticoagulants is controversial, but almost all are agreed that they do not influence the course of coronary artery disease itself. However, the drugs do reduce the incidence of deep venous thrombosis which can be as high as 40 per cent in complicated cases; the risk of pulmonary emboli is thereby decreased. The risk of systemic emboli from mural clot may also be reduced, but information on this point is sparse. In Brighton, patients are anticoagulated for the first 4 to 7 days using heparin in 5% dextrose.

Dose: for loading, 5000 units as undiluted injection;
for maintenance, 40 000 units daily for 2 days, then 35 000 units daily, subject if possible to laboratory control.

The drug should not be used in the presence of any contraindications to anticoagulants. These include old age, history of peptic ulcer, history of any bleeding tendency, pericarditis, and pervenous pacing. In the absence of a friction rub, pericarditis can be diagnosed with reasonable certainty if pain of cardiac type is exacerbated by respiration. A very abrupt onset of pain,

13

a widening of the mediastinal shadow, or the absence of major peripheral pulses all suggest the possibility of dissection which must prohibit the use of anticoagulants.

5. *Laxatives.* Patients with recent infarction should be protected as far as possible from straining at stool, and laxatives — either Senokot or mild bulk-type agents — should be administered to any patient with a tendency to constipation. Liquid paraffin should not be used either alone or in the form of an emulsion because it may interfere with the absorption of drugs.

DISORDERS OF CARDIAC RHYTHM COMPLICATING MYOCARDIAL INFARCTION

Sinus Bradycardia

Sinus bradycardia is one of the most important disorders of rhythm occurring after myocardial infarction. The word bradycardia usually implies a heart rate of less than 60 beats per minute, but as a definition it is too inflexible in the present context. A heart rate of 70 or even 80 per minute may be abnormally slow in a patient with clinical shock and hypotension; this can be considered a *relative* bradycardia, and in some circumstances it should be treated.

Sinus arrest and sino-atrial block are other related conditions in which the pacemaker activity of the sinus node is suppressed, or fails to propagate into the atria. They may be indistinguishable one from another on the surface electrocardiogram, for both are manifest by the absence of atrial activity. This may cause brief episodes of asystole (Fig. 1.2), or the control of the heart may pass to a subsidiary pacemaker (Fig. 1.3).

The two principal causes of sinus bradycardia and sino-atrial block are:

1. Increased vagal tone due to pain. Most patients have a period of bradycardia during the first hour following an infarct, but the heart rate increases as pain becomes less intense.

2. Ischaemic damage to the sino-atrial node. Bradycardia of this type occurs most commonly in patients with inferior infarction.

14

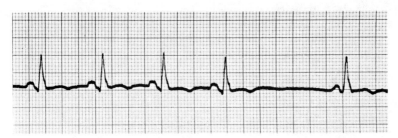

Fig. 1.2. Recent inferior ischaemia (lead II). The 5th P wave fails to appear at the expected time due to sino-atrial block, and a complete complex is lost.

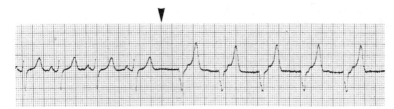

Fig. 1.3. A monitoring lead recorded from a patient with recent myocardial ischaemia. After the 4th QRS complex, the expected P wave fails to appear (arrow). The failure of the sinus pacemaker permits a subsidiary pacemaker to take control of the heart.

Sinus bradycardia can be an important complication for several reasons. First, the damaged left ventricle will be unable to compensate adequately for a slow heart rate by increasing stroke volume, and cardiac output may be reduced. Secondly, sinus bradycardia may permit the emergence of an 'escape' rhythm from an idionodal or an idioventricular pacemaker (as for sino-atrial block, Fig. 1.3). The relationship of atrial contraction to ventricular contraction is thus disturbed, and the loss of atrial boost will further reduce cardiac output, and cause an increase in atrial pressures. These adverse effects will be particularly important if the P waves fall regularly on or just after the QRS complexes, so that atrial contraction occurs against closed AV valves and propels the blood retrogradely. Thirdly, ventricular extrasystoles are more likely to occur when the basic heart

15

rate is slow; the risk of a serious ventricular arrhythmia triggered by an extrasystole is therefore greater.

Sinus bradycardia persisting after the relief of pain should be treated in any of the following circumstances:

i. if the heart rate falls below 50 per minute;
ii. if the patient has clinical evidence of a low output state;
iii. if the bradycardia is complicated by ventricular extrasystoles or other dangerous rhythm disturbances.

Atropine is the drug of choice for the treatment of sinus bradycardia or sino-atrial block. It is highly effective when the bradycardia is due entirely to increased vagal tone; in cases with ischaemic damage to the sino-atrial node the response is variable and sometimes disappointing. Because of the small risk of a brisk increase in heart rate, and also because of the transient vagotonic action of the drug, the initial dose should be 0·3 mg, followed after two or three minutes by another 0·3 mg, and if necessary by one or two doses of 0·6 mg. If the total dose of 1·8 mg is ineffective, other treatment should be used. The choice then lies between an infusion of isoprenaline 1 to 2 μg/min or atrial pacing. Atropine is one of the safest of drugs, but the high risk of acute retention of urine must be remembered, and it is strongly, contraindicated in patients with glaucoma. The dry mouth which almost invariably results from its use distresses some patients. It may cause transient but severe mental disturbances in some patients (especially the elderly), and at worst the manifestations may resemble delirium tremens.

Supraventricular Extrasystoles

This term embraces extrasystoles arising either from the atria or from the region of the AV node. Characteristically, the QRS will show the same configuration as in sinus beats, and their supraventricular origin is then beyond doubt. Unfortunately, supraventricular extrasystoles may be conducted through the ventricles aberrantly: the QRS is then widened and of a different configuration from the usual complexes. Under these circumstances, the distinction from ventricular extrasystoles may be difficult or even impossible. Aberrant conduction occurs:

16

i. if the interval between the previous beat and the extrasystole is too short to permit full recovery of the ventricular conducting pathways. The right bundle has a longer refractory period than the left, and consequently aberrant beats frequently show the pattern of right bundle-branch block (RBBB);

ii. if extrasystoles arise near the AV node but from one side of the conducting pathway; the sequence of ventricular depolarization may then be slightly modified;

iii. if the patient has a pre-existing disturbance of intraventricular conduction.

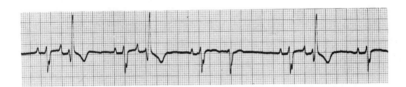

Fig. 1.4. Atrial extrasystoles conducted to the ventricles with aberration (2nd, 4th, and 8th complexes). The lead is V_1. The aberrant complexes therefore show a RBBB pattern. Each one is preceded by a P wave which is slightly more peaked than the sinus P waves. The 6th complex is also a supraventricular extrasystole which is conducted almost normally.

Extrasystoles of a wide and abnormal configuration will almost certainly be supraventricular if they are preceded by a P wave (Fig 1.4); they *may* be supraventricular if the configuration is of RBBB type and not followed by a full compensatory pause. Monitoring leads should preferably be arranged to give a pattern resembling V1 so that complexes of RBBB type can readily be recognized. But *in the context of coronary care, consider all extrasystoles with abnormally wide QRS complexes to be ventricular unless there are very good reasons for thinking otherwise.*

Supraventricular extrasystoles rarely require any specific treatment. Sometimes their appearance presages the onset of atrial fibrillation or supraventricular tachycardia; slow digitalization may therefore be indicated if a rapid arrhythmia could pose a threat to the patient.

17

Supraventricular Tachycardia

Atrial and junctional tachycardias are included under this heading, for the distinction between sites of origin is even more difficult than for extrasystoles. P waves will often be seen, but unless the beginning or the end of the rhythm abnormality is recorded there can be no certainty whether a P wave is linked to the QRS complex which follows it or which precedes it. The proximity of the P wave to one or other complex is an unreliable guide. Moreover, recent studies indicate that many supraventricular tachycardias depend upon a circus movement between the atrium and the region of the AV node; in such rhythm disturbances it is meaningless to assign a site of origin because the tachycardia does not depend upon a single ectopic pacemaker focus.

The QRS complexes of supraventricular tachycardia may be conducted normally, in which case the diagnosis is straightforward. If they are conducted aberrantly, a right bundle branch pattern is usual. The association of one P wave in fixed relationship to every QRS further supports a supraventricular origin, but even this is not fully conclusive. Again, in the context of coronary care, consider all tachycardias with abnormally wide QRS complexes to be ventricular unless there are very good reasons for thinking otherwise.

Many cases of supraventricular tachycardia will revert to sinus rhythm with carotid massage. Rarely ventricular ectopic beats which follow the breaking of a tachycardia by this manoeuvre can provoke ventricular fibrillation; special caution is necessary if digitalis toxicity is a possibility. A defibrillator should therefore be close at hand when carotid massage is attempted. If carotid massage is ineffective, the treatment depends upon the ventricular rate and upon the condition of the patient. For fast rates, more than 140 per minute, or for patients in low output states, an immediate DC shock is usually the treatment of choice; adequate anaesthesia can be obtained with intravenous diazepam. After the shock, the patient should be digitalized so that the risk of recurrence is reduced. Slower rates tend to be more difficult to revert than fast ones, but the urgency is less and digoxin alone (see p. 41) may be tried. Intravenous verapamil or practolol

18

may also be effective, but they are not free from risk. Practolol, like other β-blocking drugs, may precipitate failure and should be used with great caution if there is any evidence of impaired myocardial function. Verapamil may cause excessive slowing or asystole in a patient who has previously received a β-blocking drug, or large doses of digoxin. Lignocaine is rarely useful in supraventricular tachycardia, but it causes relatively little myocardial depression and has a brief duration of action. Lignocaine may therefore be tried before other more potent drugs which carry a higher risk of adverse effects.

Recurrent supraventricular tachycardia can usually be controlled with digoxin either alone or in combination with practolol or other antiarrhythmic drugs. In rare refractory cases rapid atrial stimulation (preferably at about 3000 impulses per minute) may be used to convert supraventricular tachycardia to atrial fibrillation in which the ventricular response will be slower (Fig. 1.5). Great care must be taken to ensure that the electrode is high in the atrium, and not in the ventricle. If specialized equipment for rapid atrial stimulation is not available, conversion to atrial fibrillation may sometimes be achieved by atrial stimulation at 10 to 20 mA and relatively slow rates presumably because some impulses fall by chance on the atrial vulnerable period. Conversion to atrial fibrillation may be particularly useful if supraventricular tachycardia is due to digitalis excess, for DC shock is hazardous in this situation. However, drug therapy is usually more appropriate.

Atrial Flutter and Atrial Tachycardia with A–V Block

Typical atrial flutter is an uncommon complication of myocardial infarction, but rapid atrial rhythms with AV block occur relatively frequently. If the block is variable and the atrial activity is of low voltage on the external ECG, the rhythm may be mistaken for atrial fibrillation. This is not usually an important error because DC shock or digoxin are likely to be effective for both. DC shock should be avoided if a high degree of AV block is present spontaneously, with a relatively slow ventricular rate.

19

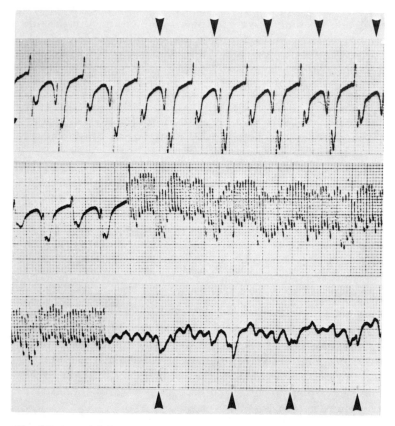

Fig. 1.5. An atrial electrogram, paper speed 50 mm/sec. Atrial tachycardia (or flutter) with 2:1 A–V block, converted to atrial fibrillation. Top strip: each sharp deflection, with a single spike above and bifid deflection below, represents a P wave. The alternating undulation results from widened QRS complexes at half the atrial rate (arrows). Middle strip: start of rapid atrial stimulation at 3000 per minute. Bottom strip: when rapid stimulation ceases, the pattern shows atrial fibrillation with QRS complexes just discernible (arrows). Atrial fibrillation seen in an atrial electrogram may resemble ventricular fibrillation on an external electrogram.

Atrial Fibrillation

This common rhythm disturbance presents little diagnostic difficulty. However, the disparity in R–R intervals may be

20

responsible for variation in patterns of intraventricular conduction, and aberration is particularly likely to occur in a complex terminating a short interval which has followed a long one. Such aberrant complexes are sometimes mistaken for ventricular extrasystoles, and suppressant drugs are then given unnecessarily.

For cases in which impaired AV conductivity causes a ventricular response of less than 100 per minute, treatment is unnecessary, and indeed may be unwise. If the ventricular rate is more than 130 per minute, DC shock is usually indicated; for even if the patient's condition is satisfactory the greater metabolic demands of a rapid heart rate may increase the zone of necrosis in an ischaemic area. For rates between 100 and 130 per minute, the usual treatment is digitalization, but if the patient has a critical low output state attempted conversion to sinus rhythm with a DC shock is mandatory. In some instances the ventricular response to atrial fibrillation is rapid even with adequate digitalization. Verapamil may then cautiously be used to slow the rate. Practolol is more dangerous because of the greater risk of inducing severe failure, but the effect can be beneficial if the rate response outweighs the impairment of contractility. Very small doses (e.g. 2 mg i.v.) should be given in the first instance, and incremented only if the response is favourable.

Atrioventricular Block and Asystole

Complete AV block occurs in up to 8 per cent of patients with acute myocardial infarction who are admitted to hospital. The clinical and electrocardiographic features of this important complication depend upon the site of the infarct which caused the block.

In most instances the infarction is inferior resulting from an occlusion in the right coronary artery or occasionally in a dominant left circumflex artery. Block usually occurs as a result of oedema and inflammation around the AV node, without actual destruction of conduction tissue. Complete AV block occurring at this level is typically preceded by prolongation of the PR interval, and later by second-degree block of the Wenckebach type. When complete block supervenes, lower junctional tissue within the conduction system takes over pace-maker function, and in most patients the QRS complexes retain a configuration similar to that of previously conducted beats, with a ventricular rate usually in the range 40 to 80 beats per minute (Fig. 1.6). Asystole is unlikely to occur because junctional pacemakers provide a reliable escape mechanism. The mortality is only slightly higher than that of inferior infarction not complicated by block.

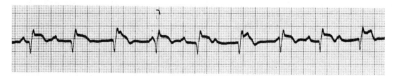

Fig. 1.6. Recent inferior myocardial infarction (lead II) with complete heart block and an accelerated junctional rhythm. In this case the ventricular rate was somewhat faster than usual at 88 per minute.

In some cases of inferior infarction a junctional pacemaker accelerates to a rate more rapid than that of the sinus mechanism. AV dissociation is then inevitable (Fig. 1.7) unless the junctional pacemaker also captures the atrium by retrograde activation. The phenomenon does *not* imply antegrade AV block which can be diagnosed only when the atrial rate is *faster* than the ventricular rate.

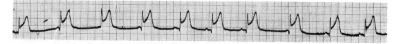

Fig. 1.7. Recent inferior myocardial infraction (lead II). The atrial rate is relatively slow, and showing marked sinus arrhythmia. When the P–P intervals are long, the junctional pacemaker takes over at its own intrinsic rate of 53 per minute, causing AV dissociation (2nd, 3rd, 4th, 8th, and 9th complexes). There is no heart block, and the faster P waves do conduct normally (1st, 5th, 6th, 7th, and 10th complexes).

The sequence of events is quite different in cases of anterior infarction. An occlusion usually in the anterior descending branch of the left coronary artery causes necrosis in the left ventricle and anterior part of the interventricular septum remote from the AV node. Block occurs only if both bundle-branches are involved, and for this to happen the area of muscle damage

22

must be extensive. Many patients have evidence of previous inferior infarction. Prolongation of the PR interval is not usually seen: in the bundle-branches, impulses tend either to be conducted without delay or be blocked completely. However, complete block may be heralded by the onset of right or left bundle-branch block. The sudden development of left axis deviation indicates a conduction defect in the superior division of the left bundle-branch; right bundle-branch block plus left axis deviation is therefore a particularly important warning sign for it indicates that failure of impulse transmission has occurred in two of the three conducting pathways. If second-degree block does occur it is of Mobitz type II rather than Wenckebach type, in which one or more P waves abruptly fail to conduct to the ventricles (Fig. 1.8). After the development of complete heart block of this type, any escape rhythm must be idioventricular. The QRS complexes are therefore wide and of abnormal configuration. Idioventricular pacemakers are usually slow, sometimes irregular, and always unreliable. Adams—Stokes attacks or sudden death may occur at any time as a result of asystole or asystole followed by ventricular fibrillation.

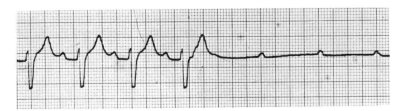

Fig. 1.8. An electrocardiogram (lead II) illustrating Mobitz type II second degree AV block. The patient had had a recent anterior myocardial infarction; he developed right bundle branch block and left axis deviation. Conduction to the ventricles failed abruptly for several seconds. Although the PR interval had been 0·24 second, no further prolongation occurred before the period of asystole.

Some cases of AV block with *inferior* infarction have a satisfactory heart rate and do not require treatment. Specific therapy is indicated if the patient's condition suggests serious impairment of cardiac output or if the spontaneous rate is less than 50 per minute. Atropine should be given intravenously, starting with 0·6 mg but increasing the dose if necessary to a maximum of 1·8 mg. This can be repeated every 4 to 6 hours. If atropine is ineffective, isoprenaline should be given by continuous intravenous infusion, preferably using an accurate drip counter or pump to maintain a constant dose rate of 1 to 4 μg per minute. 2·5 mg isoprenaline dissolved in 500 ml isotonic dextrose produces a suitable concentration for infusion. The indications for pacing are usually relative, and include such factors as inadequate response to drug therapy, abnormal intraventricular conduction suggesting an idioventricular rather than a junctional escape rhythm, congestive heart failure, and recurrent ventricular arrhythmias. Very rarely, asystole does occur and even a brief episode constitutes an absolute indication for pacing.

Pacing is always mandatory for complete AV block in *anterior* infarction, for isoprenaline is relatively ineffective and atropine totally ineffective as means of increasing heart rate. Unfortunately, even with the reduced risk of asystole and the improved cardiac output which may accrue, the mortality remains extremely high. This is in part a reflection of the extensive muscle necrosis which is present in these patients, and most of those who are successfully paced die of cardiogenic shock. Many more patients die before electrical pacing can be established. The very important differences in complete heart block complicating inferior infarction and anterior infarction are summarized in Table I.

Complete absence of myocardial activity (asystole) usually indicates massive heart damage except when it occurs as a transient phenomenon, or when it is due to a severe metabolic disturbance. Treatment is therefore relatively ineffective and the prognosis is grave. Rarely, persistent asystole may result from failure of a subsidiary pacemaker to emerge in cases of bilateral bundle-branch block without severe muscle damage. In such cases, the heart can sometimes be 'paced' as an emergency measure by light blows to the praecordium: if this results in an effective output it is preferable to external cardiac massage. An effective spontaneous heartbeat may also be restored by an intravenous bolus of 10 ml 10% calcium chloride or by an isoprenaline infusion. The dose of isoprenaline in this situation may vary from the conventional 2 μg per minute to massive doses up to 40 μg per minute which must be curtailed

24

TABLE I

	Inferior Infarction	*Anterior Infarction*
Site of block	AV node	bundle-branches
Premonitory signs	prolongation of PR interval, Wenckebach AV block	development of RBBB, LAD, or LBBB
Subsidiary pacemakers:		
site	above bifurcation of bundle of His (junctional)	below bifurcation of bundle of His (idioventricular)
QRS	may be narrow	usually widened
rate	40–80 per minute	20–40 per minute
reliability	excellent	poor
Artificial pacing	usually unnecessary	mandatory
Immediate prognosis	reasonably good	grave
Recovery of conduction in survivors	invariable	usual
Late asystole	never	probably common

immediately some response is achieved. These doses are conveniently obtained by mixing 2·5 mg isoprenaline in 500 ml of dextrose and setting the drip rate from 10 to 200 drips per minute. Note that the drip tubing must be flushed through with the solution before it is connected to the patient. Pacing must be initiated as soon as possible.

Insertion of pacemaker electrode

Several venous routes have been recommended for the introduction of pacing electrodes, and all have disadvantages. The easiest route is from a medial antecubital vein, but arm movements may subsequently dislodge the tip of the electrode. Binding the arm to the chest wall obviates this difficulty at the cost of inconvenience to the patient. The external jugular route provides a stable electrode position, though entry into the vein and manipulation from this site are slightly more difficult. The percutaneous subclavian route is very satisfactory in skilled hands. When the tip is correctly positioned, preferably in the apex of the right ventricle, only a gentle curve of electrode

25

should be visible in the atrium (Fig. 9.1), for a redundant loop will increase the risk of penetration of the myocardium or permit dislodgement of the tip into the pulmonary artery. The

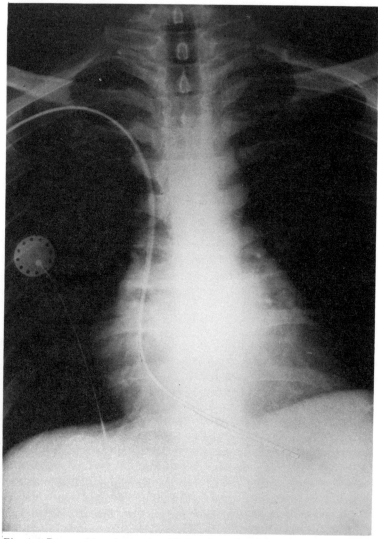

Fig. 1.9. Pacemaking electrode with the tip in the right ventricle (retouched for clarity). Only a gentle curve, without any redundant loop, is seen within the right atrium. (The right diaghragm is high and obscuring part of the heart shadow.)

position of the electrode tip is satisfactory only if the threshold for pacing is low, preferably less than 1 volt, and remains stable during deep inspiration. Treatment with isoprenaline should be discontinued during manipulation of the electrode, and a DC defibrillator must be ready for immediate use because ventricular fibrillation is an occasional complication of the procedure.

If screening facilities are not available, a fine Teflon-coated platinum-tipped stainless steel wire electrode can be introduced through a small catheter extending to the superior vena cava. The electrode can be manoeuvred into the ventricle by monitoring an intracardiac electrogram recorded from its tip; a striking change in the tracing occurs as soon as the tricuspid valve is traversed (Fig. 1.10).

It is important, of course, that the input of any mains electrocardiograph should be isolated if intracavity electrograms are to be recorded. Much of the older equipment at present in use

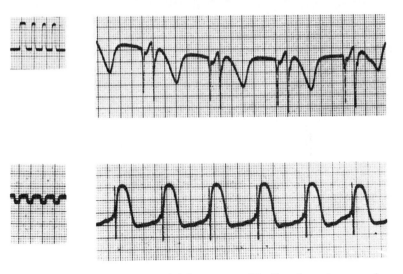

Fig. 1.10. Top strip: typical atrial electrogram. The first sharp downward deflection is the P wave, and the second is the QRS. The configuration of both deflections in the atrium varies considerably depending upon the site of the electrode, and also varies from patient to patient. Lower strip (note ¼ sensitivity): typical ventricular electrogram. The P wave can no longer be discerned. The electrode is in contact with the endocardium, giving rise to a markedly elevated ST segment resembling a current of injury.

27

would be unsuitable for this purpose. Fine electrodes can also be used for atrial pacing to increase heart rate in patients with normal conduction who have refractory arrhythmias or brady-cardia. Although these techniques cause little disturbance to the patient, they do require considerable expertise and should not be undertaken lightly by those without special training.

The external pacemaker

The unit used for a patient with myocardial infarction should always be of the demand type to reduce the risk of ven-tricular fibrillation as a result of competition between paced beats and spontaneous beats. This is important even in cases of complete block, for in survivors AV conduction almost always recovers, and the threshold for the electrical induction of ventricular fibrillation is reduced. The pacemaker unit is set at approximately twice the output necessary to capture the ventricle, to allow for small changes in stimulating threshold. This should be checked 4-hourly and the output reset if necessary. Small increases in threshold are common, but a sudden change implies displacement of the electrode or penetration of the myocardium. An unnecessarily high output setting increases the risk of pacemaker-induced arrhythmias. Ideally, a ventricular electrogram should be recorded from the pacing electrode before it is secured to ensure that the signal is stable and also strong enough to inhibit the demand pacemaker, because low intracardiac potentials may occur in patients with myocardial infarction. A signal of 2·0 mV is adequate for most units. There is no general agreement on the length of time for which the demand pacemaker should be left in place following recovery of AV conduction. Some patients with anterior infarction die from a recurrence of asystole late in the course of their hospital admission. If pacing has been uncomplicated, the unit should probably be left connected, but inactive at a rate setting below that of the sinus rate, for at least a week after conduction has returned. This precaution is, of course, unnecessary in most of the patients with inferior infarction who require pacing for one of the indications discussed above.

The rate at which the ventricular pacemaker is set depends upon the degree of impairment of the circulation and upon the stability of the paced rhythm. Cardiac output is enhanced by ventricular pacing in myocardial infarction with AV block, and within limits will continue to improve as rate is increased. On the other hand, myocardial oxygen requirement becomes progressively greater with faster rates. In practice, pacing rates of 60 to 100 beats a minute are usually chosen, but faster rates may be necessary to help counteract shock or to suppress ventricular arrhythmias.

A reliable estimate of the effect of artificial pacing on the mortality rate in myocardial infarction has never been obtained. If the problem were to be oversimplified for the sake of emphasis, one could say that in patients with inferior infarction and AV block, pacing is usually unnecessary; for patients with anterior infarction and block it is usually futile because the mortality is very high with or without treatment. In fact some patients with inferior infarction *do* require pacing, and some paced patients with anterior infarction and block *do* survive. Moreover, the technique can be valuable in the control of refractory tachyarrhythmias and sinus bradycardia. The technique is not free from risk even in experienced hands, and so the selection of patients for this form of treatment must be made with care. There is no doubt that ventricular pacing does have a small but important role in the management of myocardial infarction, and that overall it has a favourable effect upon prognosis.

Ventricular Extrasystoles
The configuration of extrasystoles arising in the ventricles depends upon the site of the ectopic focus. This is usually remote from the bundle of His; the pattern of depolarization is therefore abnormal and the QRS complex is widened and bizarre in shape. The shape will resemble that of right bundle-branch block if the focus is in the left ventricle, and left bundle-branch block if the focus is on the right. A minority of ventricular extrasystoles arise in the interventricular septum above the bifurcation of the bundle, and resemble conducted beats. The distinction from junctional complexes is therefore not hard and fast, especially since higher junctional ectopics may show aberrant conduction (p. 16). Even very wide complexes may be supraventricular in origin if the patient has pre-existing bundle-branch block or if a major part of the conducting system is still

29

refractory when the extrasystole is transmitted into the
ventricles. Many supraventricular extrasystoles conducted with
marked aberration have the following characteristics:

  i. a right bundle-branch block pattern with:

  ii. an RSR^1 pattern in V_1 rather than qR;

  iii. less than a full compensatory pause;

  iv. if of atrial or high junctional origin, they will be preceded by
a P wave.

However, the distinction cannot usually be made with any
certainty, and it is preferable to assume that extrasystoles are
ventricular whenever doubt exists.

Ventricular extrasystoles cause little functional disturbance,
but they have a sinister connotation, especially in relationship
to acute myocardial ischaemia, because they may presage ventricular tachycardia and ventricular fibrillation. Unfortunately,
ventricular fibrillation can occur in patients who have had few
or even no 'warning' extrasystoles, and in others frequent extrasystoles may occur without further complications. Moreover,
some recent evidence suggests that the extrasystoles which occur
in the first hour or two after infarction, when the risk of fibrillation is high, are more difficult to suppress than those which
occur late in the course of the illness. For these reasons, the risk
of ventricular fibrillation cannot easily be abolished by control
of extrasystoles in the Coronary Care Unit, but its incidence can
be reduced. Suppressive treatment should be given in the following circumstances:

  i. if ventricular extrasystoles are occurring frequently, perhaps
more than 5 per minute;

  ii. if extrasystoles occur consecutively (two in a row are much
more than twice as 'evil' as a single one);

  iii. if the coupling intervals are short or the T waves of the
preceding beats are prolonged so that the extrasystoles occur
near the peak of the T waves ('vulnerable period');

  iv. if the ventricular extrasystoles are 'multiform', i.e. they vary
in shape and may therefore arise from more than one focus;

  v. if the patient has already experienced ventricular tachycardia
or fibrillation.

Although multiform extrasystoles are ominous in that they
indicate considerable electrical instability, they do not always

arise from different foci. Sometimes a single focus may conduct by varying pathways (particularly if the R—R intervals are changing); in other instances late ventricular extrasystoles may 'fuse' with conducted beats producing QRS complexes of a hybrid type (Fig. 1.11). The shape of the extrasystoles are of importance in one more respect; in general, wide complexes are more likely to be dangerous than narrow ones which resemble conducted beats.

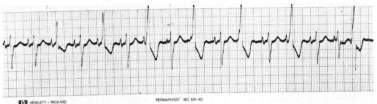

HEWLETT · PACKARD   PERMAPAPER® NO. 651-40

Fig. 1.11. Ventricular extrasystoles and sinus tachycardia. The 3rd, 5th, 7th, 9th, and 11th complexes show a varying relationship between extrasystoles and P waves. When the extrasystole occurs relatively late, normal depolarization of the ventricle has already started, and a 'fused' beat results (part normally-conducted and part extrasystolic). The 11th complex is the purest extrasystole in the strip, and the others show intermediate forms.

The choice of treatment for suppressing ventricular extra-systoles depends upon the rate of the dominant rhythm. A heart rate which is disproportionately slow for the haemodynamic state of the patient is common after myocardial infarction, and bradycardia favours the emergence of ectopic pacemakers. In such cases, 0·3 mg atropine should be given intravenously, followed if necessary by further doses to a maximum of 1·8 mg. In the absence of bradycardia, lignocaine should be used for the suppression of extrasystoles. This should be given in an initial dose of 75 to 100 mg intravenously over two or three minutes, followed by an infusion of 2 to 4 mg per minute, but the dose should be reduced in the presence of known liver disease or critical low output states (Fig. 1.12). A constant rate infusion pump is recommended to prevent large doses inadvertently run-ning in rapidly. Five per cent dextrose is a suitable diluent for lignocaine. Phenytoin, bretylium, and procainamide are appro-priate drugs to use if lignocaine is ineffective, and β-blocking agents may also be used if myocardial function is not seriously impaired. However, one must resist the temptation of hazarding

31

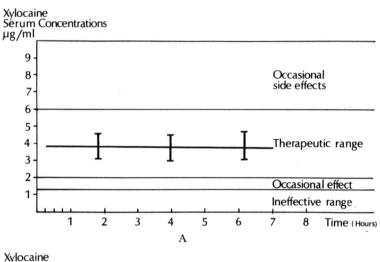

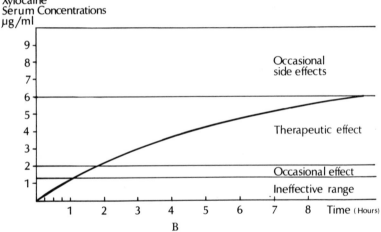

Fig. 1.12. The results of Lignocaine ('Xylocaine') infusion, serum concentrations plotted against time. A: the mean results of 3 mg/min in patients with normal hepatic function. B: an example of rising plasma concentration during an infusion of 3 mg/min in a patient with poor hepatic function. These are idealized curves based upon pooled data provided by Astra Chemicals Ltd.

the patient's life by large doses of suppressant drugs in the absence of any indication that the extrasystoles are truly dangerous. How far to insist on suppression in any individual patient is a matter for fine judgement.

Ventricular Tachycardia

This rhythm is thought to arise from the repetitive firing of an abnormal focus within the ventricles, and therefore represents a succession of consecutive ventricular extrasystoles. By general usage, a run of three or more extrasystoles should be called a tachycardia, provided, of course, the rate is greater than 100 per minute. Although ventricular tachycardia is characterized by bizarre widened QRS complexes, the diagnosis is not straight-forward, for supraventricular tachycardia may also have widened complexes if the patient has pre-existing bundle-branch block, or if the conduction is aberrant due to incomplete recovery of the conducting pathways between each depolarization. A supra-ventricular origin should be suspected:

i. if the QRS has a right bundle-branch block pattern (but RSR^1, not qR in V$_1$), and
ii. in the *absence* of atrial activity at a different rate and inde-pendent of QRS complexes.

However, the distinction cannot be made with certainty at the bedside, for even a tachycardia which *does* have independent P waves may be junctional with a retrograde V—A block. The best available indication of a ventricular origin is the presence of 'fusion' due to interference from conducted supraventricular beats (see p. 31 and Fig. 1.11). The usual rule obtains: in the presence of recent ischaemia it is safer to assume a ventricular origin whenever reasonable doubt exists.

Ventricular tachycardia is an ominous complication. If the rate is fast the cardiac output may fall, and if this reaches critically low levels a metabolic acidosis may cause further instability of rhythm. Moreover, a rapid heart rate increases the myocardial demands for oxygen, and areas of ischaemic muscle which had been capable of recovery may become necrosed. An even greater danger is the possible progression of ventricular tachycardia to ventricular fibrillation, and here, too, the rate is important. Slower ventricular rhythms tend to be more stable than rapid ones, and the most sinister of all is an accelerating tachycardia which often breaks down into fibrillation within seconds.

One of the prime aims of coronary care units is to prevent

ventricular tachycardia by suppressing any dangerous ectopic focus, but this is an ideal which cannot always be attained. When ventricular tachycardia occurs, treatment is mandatory. The drug regime is the same as that for ventricular extrasystoles: lignocaine is the agent of choice, but phenytoin, bretylium, procainamide, and (with reservations) β-blocking drugs may be used if lignocaine is known to be ineffective. If the patient's condition is poor, or if the rate is seen to be accelerating, or if the rhythm has not responded within a few minutes to drug therapy the patient should be given a DC shock after premedication with intravenous diazepam.

Problems arise in dealing with recurrent ventricular tachycardia. If possible, suppression should be achieved with drugs; procainamide and bretylium are probably the most successful for this purpose. Drug therapy should not be abandoned without a trial of magnesium sulphate. An alternative form of treatment is by rapid ventricular pacing. Ectopic foci are more likely to emerge with a relatively slow basic rhythm than with a fast one, and virtually all ectopic foci can be suppressed if the basic rhythm is fast enough. The rate which is necessary to attain control varies from one instance to another but frequently pacing at an acceptable rate will stabilize the rhythm. Disadvantages of the technique include the need for expertise and screening facilities, the small inherent dangers of electrical pacing in myocardial infarction, and the increased oxygen requirement of the myocardium at higher sustained rates of contraction. As a last resort, patients with recurrent ventricular tachycardia may require frequent shocks. This can cause great distress to a conscious patient, and opiates should therefore be used liberally. Under these circumstances, respiration is best maintained by artificial ventilation.

Slow Idioventricular Rhythm

This must be distinguished from ventricular tachycardia. It is very common in the first hours after myocardial infarction, often appearing as an 'escape rhythm' secondary to sinus bradycardia or sino-atrial block (Fig. 1.3, p. 15) or occasionally to atrioventricular block. Such rhythms are usually transient and benign. The correct treatment is *not* suppression of the

34

ectopic focus for this may lead to dangerous bradycardia or even asystole. Atropine may be used to counter sinus bradycardia and so permit the re-emergence of the dominant pacemaker. In the presence of atrioventricular block, an escape rhythm with a widened QRS is usually accepted as an indication for electrical pacing.

Ventricular Fibrillation

The introduction in recent years of external cardiac massage and electrical defibrillation have transformed ventricular fibrillation from an inevitable terminal event into a potentially remediable medical emergency. Drug therapy also has a place in the management of circulatory arrest but the efficacy of the agents in common use is difficult to evaluate, and many will doubtless be superseded.

The speed with which resuscitative procedures are instituted is critical for two reasons: first, because cerebral necrosis will occur after two to four minutes of circulatory arrest, and secondly because the likelihood of successful restoration of an effective circulation diminishes rapidly as the seconds pass by. Many patients who suffer unexpected ventricular fibrillation are young or middle-aged and do not necessarily have severely impaired myocardial function. Moreover, a successful outcome may be followed by many years of healthy life. For these reasons it is mandatory for every general hospital to have a highly organized and well-drilled system for dealing with this, the most dire of all medical emergencies.

The organization of the cardiac arrest procedure is of equal importance to the expertise of the medical personnel. An easily dialled (preferably single figure) number should command immediate priority at the hospital switchboard. Ideally, an anaesthetist and at least one other doctor should be available on an 'emergency' bleep; if a 2-tone system is not used, an arrest call can be characterized in some more simple manner. The emergency box present in the Coronary Care Unit and in every ward should contain a *minimum* of essential equipment, and only those drugs which have to be on hand within a minute or so. The boxes should be checked at least weekly, and preferably by the same person throughout the hospital. Special attention has to be given to connections for anaesthetic equipment because of the lack of standardization in this field. If defibrillators and oscilloscopes are not available in all wards, they should be placed strategically so that they can be moved without delay, particularly to those wards admitting coronary patients. It may be preferable for a hospital porter to carry a bleep and to be part of the arrest 'team'; only one or two nurses may be in the ward and they should be at the bedside and not searching for equipment elsewhere. The equipment itself should be portable, and preferably battery-operated. It must be checked frequently as a routine and always after use. Portable combined defibrillator-oscilloscopes are now becoming available, and those which use the defibrillation paddles to receive the ECG signal are particularly convenient for use outside high dependency areas. The defibrillator should reach maximum charge rapidly, certainly within 20 seconds. Unfortunately, one of the models currently in common use depends upon a battery of 24 1·5 V cells, the specification of which cannot be guaranteed; a charge-time as long as 2 minutes may be observed, and this is unsuitable for emergency situations.* Any paste manufactured for use with electrocardiographs is suitable for contact between the defibrillator paddles and the patient; KY jelly should *not* be used because it contains no electrolyte and therefore reduces effective current flow. Considerable attention should be paid to the elimination of even minor problems: I have found it of great value to have a form completed after every arrest call requesting details of any delays or difficulties which were observed during the procedure.

When a cardiac arrest occurs outside a high dependency area, the patient is unlikely to be receiving constant electrocardiographic monitoring. The distinction between ventricular fibrillation and asystole cannot be made clinically, but a sharp blow to the praecordium is always appropriate and has a small chance of restoring coordinated contraction. If a defibrillator is available, a single DC shock may reasonably be given before an electrocardiogram is available, for this may avoid delay in the treatment of fibrillation and be ineffective but harmless in asystole.

---

* Cardiac Recorders Ltd. have introduced a rechargeable nickel-cadmium cell as an alternative to a battery of 1·5 V cells. This has a charge-time of approximately 12 seconds. The modification can readily be made to existing defibrillators.

It most instances the first responsibility will fall to nurses trained only in the ABC of emergency resuscitation (*A*irway to be cleared, *B*reathing (ventilation) to be initiated, *C*ardiac compression to be performed). The major pitfalls in these procedures are well known and must be stressed during instruction: failure to extend the neck sufficiently to achieve a patent airway, the practical difficulties of inflating the patient's lungs, the ineffective use of external massage on a well-sprung hospital bed.

The delay in resuscitation in a general ward almost inevitably implies respiratory as well as cardiac arrest and intubation is then an early priority. Provided ventilation and cardiac compression are effective, patients may rarely survive up to an hour without spontaneous heart action before more definitive measures can be instituted.

With the increasing availability of high dependency areas, many patients suffering cardiac arrest have highly skilled personnel close at hand. Little time should be wasted in recognizing the emergency, and constant electrocardiographic monitoring permits an immediate distinction between ventricular fibrillation and asystole. The definitive treatment of ventricular fibrillation is defibrillation, and the quicker the shock is delivered the better the prospects for a successful outcome. It follows that senior nurses in Coronary Care Units, in intensive care units, and even in general medical wards should be trained in the safe use of defibrillators and not restricted to performing external massage and artificial ventilation. These latter procedures must, of course, be instituted for any but the briefest period of circulatory arrest, and maintained as far as is practicable until an effective circulation is restored.

The defibrillator paddles should be placed one on the front of the praecordium and the other well to the left (Fig. 1.13); if a flat paddle is available the second position should be under the left shoulder blade. Monitoring electrodes and dressings must be avoided. Neither the operator nor any other attendant should be touching the patient or bed when the shock is delivered. The electrode paste should cover the area of skin in contact with the paddles, but if it flows from one paddle position to the other the current will arc dangerously and ineffectively across the surface of the chest. The paste should be kept away from the

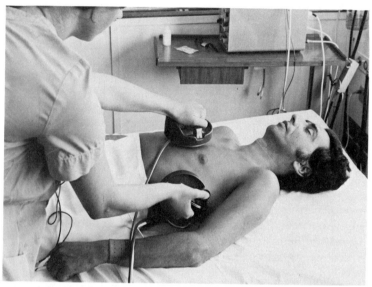

Fig. 1.13. The usual positions for defibrillating electrodes.

upper surface of the paddles and from the operator's hands to avoid danger to himself. A charge of 200 joules may be used for the first shock if the patient has been in ventricular fibrillation for less than 30 seconds. Otherwise, it is preferable to use the maximum charge of 400 joules to avoid dangerous delay.

Successful defibrillation is followed by a period of asystole which varies in duration. If QRS complexes do not appear on the monitoring oscilloscope within a few seconds, the heart may be stimulated by one or, if necessary, by a succession of light blows to the praecordium. Should this manoeuvre be unsuccessful, full external cardiac massage and artificial ventilation must be recommenced without delay. Cardiac massage is also essential as an interim measure until coordinated rhythm is accompanied by a palpable pulse, for effective spontaneous contraction may lag behind the restoration of electrical depolarization.

If defibrillation is rapidly effective and the period of circulatory arrest was brief, no further treatment is necessary except for the initiation or augmentation of a prophylactic drug regime (see below). Unfortunately, defibrillation is not always successful in the first instance, especially if delay has occurred between the onset of the arrhythmia and attempts at resuscitation. This

difficulty is due in part to metabolic acidosis which builds up
rapidly during circulatory arrest, and must be countered with an
infusion of sodium bicarbonate. The immediate dose is 50–100
mEq, but for prolonged periods of arrest an additional dose
should be given according to the formula:

mEq sodium bicarbonate = 1/10 X period of arrest in minutes
X patient's weight in kg.

Solutions containing 1 mEq per ml (8·4%) are conveniently
small in volume. In general the tendency is to use too much
bicarbonate, and promote both alkalosis and sodium overload,
a hazard which has been exacerbated by the commercial availability of 'polyfusors' containing 500 mEq. In moments of
emergency, it is impractical to give a measured dose from these
containers, which are therefore too dangerous to recommend.
Arterial pH and base deficit should be checked as soon as an
effective circulation has been restored and any residual base
deficit corrected.

Defibrillation may be unsuccessful even after the correction
of acidosis. The fibrillation waveform offers some guide to subsequent therapy. An intravenous injection of 10 ml 1 : 10 000
adrenaline may coarsen fine fibrillation and render it more
responsive. If it is already coarse, the following drugs may prove
effective: lignocaine 100 mg, bretylium tosylate 300 mg (by
slow intravenous injection, preferably diluted in isotonic
dextrose), phenytoin 100 to 200 mg, magnesium sulphate
10 ml 50% solution. Injections should be as central as practicable, and sufficient time allowed for them to reach the heart
during the sluggish circulation engendered by cardiac massage.
The intracardiac route is not recommended. Again, it must be
emphasized that suppressant drugs must be used as sparingly as
possible for they all impair myocardial contractility. With the
measures outlined above, the heart can almost always be defibrillated, but effective cardiac contraction after defibrillation is
much more difficult to achieve when attempts at resuscitation
have been prolonged. The failure to obtain palpable peripheral
pulses from coordinated rhythm even after the circulation has
been supported for five to ten minutes by external massage is
an ominous sign: 10 ml of 10% calcium chloride may rarely be
effective at this stage, and an isoprenaline infusion may be used
as a desperate measure.

39

After successful defibrillation an infusion of lignocaine (2 to 4 mg per minute) may provide some measure of protection against recurrence. Our own practice is to substitute oral procainamide as soon as possible, with an initial dose of 375 mg every 3 hours. Laboratory control is necessary to maintain blood levels of 4 to 8 μg per ml. This regime is continued for 4 weeks. Recent evidence suggests that patients with recurrent episodes of fibrillation may be stabilized by bretylium tosylate (300 to 600 mg by slow i.v. infusion followed by 300 mg i.m. 8 hourly). Alternatively, the ventricle may be paced above the spontaneous rate: in favourable cases complete suppression may be attained without the need for unacceptably rapid rates.

Any prolonged period of circulatory arrest will cause cerebral oedema which further reduces cerebral blood flow. One hundred ml 10% mannitol followed by 8 mg dexamethasone intravenously helps to counter this chain of events and reduce the degree of cerebral damage.

The treatment of cardiac arrest provides a challenge because the overall survival rate is poor even in cases without severe myocardial damage. This is especially true outside high dependency areas. There can be no room for complacency because this unsatisfactory situation can almost certainly be improved by detailed attention to the organization of cardiac arrest procedures.

A summary of the treatment of arrhythmias complicating myocardial infarction is shown in Table II.

OTHER MAJOR COMPLICATIONS OF ACUTE MYOCARDIAL INFARCTION

Heart Failure

The myocardial damage resulting from ischaemic heart disease occurs principally in the left ventricle. Left-sided heart failure is therefore a relatively common complication of acute myocardial infarction, and is due to a disturbance of the fine balance which normally exists between the two sides of the heart. It may be manifest only by slight pulmonary congestion, or at the other end of the spectrum by fatal acute pulmonary oedema.

Infarction of the right ventricle is usually restricted to the

TABLE II

Sinus bradycardia	may require no treatment atropine 0·3 to 1·8 mg isoprenaline 1 to 2 μg/min atrial pacing
Supraventricular extrasystoles	usually no treatment

Supraventricular
tachycardias
	carotid massage (N.B. dangers if digitalis-induced)
	DC shock
	digoxin: if i.v. loading dose required, not usually
	    faster than 1·5 mg infused over 3 to 4 hours
	lignocaine 100 mg. Safe but often ineffective
	rarely practolol 2 to 10 mg or verapamil
	    2·5 to 10 mg (N.B. dangers)
	rapid atrial stimulation (p. 19) for refractory
	    severe cases

Atrial flutter or Atrial tachycardia with A—V block	DC shock digoxin may require no treatment if ventricular response is slow

Atrial fibrillation	ventricular rate < 100/min: usually no treatment.
	ventricular rate 100—130/min, general condition
	    good: digoxin
	ventricular rate 100—130/min, with low output
	    state: DC shock
	ventricular rate > 130/min: DC shock
	practolol and verapamil may also be used in
	    conjunction with digoxin for refractory cases,
	    but not free from risk

Complete A—V block
(see also Table I
p. 25)
	with inferior infarction: may require no treatment
	atropine 0·6 to 1·8 mg i.v., repeated 4 to 6 hourly
	    as necessary
	isoprenaline infusion 1—4 μg/min
	with anterior infarction: pervenous electrical
	    pacing

Table II (*contd.*)

Asystole	external cardiac massage pervenous electrical pacing if practicable calcium chloride 10 ml 10% solution adrenaline 10 to 50 ml 1 : 10 000 solution isoprenaline infusion 2 to 40 μg/min (massive doses curtailed as soon as possible!)

Ventricular extrasystoles	may require no treatment (and N.B. extrasystoles
	    may be preferable to drug-induced myocardial
	    depression!)
	with bradycardia: atropine 0·3 to 1·8 mg
	without bradycardia: lignocaine 75 to 100 mg
	    bolus over 2 mins followed by infusion 2—4
	    mg/min
	bretylium tosylate 300 to 600 mg in 100 ml
	    dextrose i.v. + 300 mg i.m. 8-hourly in *serious*
	    refractory cases, or:
	phenytoin 50 to 200 mg 4-hourly by central i.v.
	    injection (scleroses veins)
	(rarely procainamide, β blocking agents, or
	    magnesium sulphate)

Idioventricular or junctional rhythm	may require no treatment atropine 0·3 to 1·8 mg to restore sinus dominance
Ventricular tachycardia	drugs as for ventricular extrasystoles with rapid or accelerating rhythm, or in low out- put states: DC shock ventricular pacing for refractory cases

Ventricular fibrillation	DC shock
	use sodium bicarbonate 50 to 100 mEq + mEq
	    calculated by (1/10 X period of arrest in mins
	    X patient's weight in kg)
	for refractory or recurrent cases use drugs as for
	    ventricular extrasystoles, and if necessary rapid
	    ventricular pacing

septum, but minor damage to the free wall may occur with occlusions of the right coronary artery. Significant elevation of the jugular venous pressure reflecting right ventricular dysfunction is therefore more common with inferior myocardial infarction following right coronary occlusion than with infarcts of other types. Frank right-sided failure does, of course, occur with chronic ischaemic heart disease, but in acute myocardial infarction only left-sided failure presents serious problems of management.

The internal jugular vein acts as a manometer for accurate clinical assessment of right-sided filling pressure, but no such convenient measure of left-sided function is readily accessible. The recognition of florid pulmonary oedema is easy, but lesser degrees of left ventricular dysfunction can be diagnosed only by rather subtle physical signs and by special investigations. Sinus tachycardia disproportionate to any hypotension is very suggestive of heart failure, but may not be present in the following circumstances: during the early post-infarction phase of excess vagal tone, with inferior infarction causing ischaemia of the sino-atrial node, in elderly patients with sinus node disease, and after administration of β-adrenergic blocking agents. Another clue is given by a 'triple rhythm', the presence of the early diastolic third sound of rapid ventricular filling or the late diastolic fourth sound caused by atrial contraction. Both of these signs signify disordered relaxation or altered compliance of the left ventricle. These 'sounds' are of low frequency, and may be better felt than heard. Reversed splitting of the second heart sound is said to occur with severe impairment of left ventricular function but is rare except with left bundle-branch block or during the acute stages of infarction. The presence of basal crepitations is of very limited value for crepitations occur frequently in the absence of heart disease (especially in the elderly) and may not be present even with severe left ventricular failure.

A portable radiograph can provide an excellent guide to the degree of impairment of left ventricular function provided the quality of the picture permits inspection of the lung vasculature. It should be an essential part of the initial assessment of the patient with recent infarction. The film should be taken with the patient sitting, not supine. In the upright position the upper lobe pulmonary veins (which usually lie lateral to the corresponding arteries) are normally barely visible; but with increasing elevation of pulmonary venous pressure the veins become prominent and ultimately even wider than the arteries. The term pulmonary congestion can be used to signify this change in the appearance of the vessels. When the mean pulmonary venous pressure exceeds about 25 mm Hg, pulmonary congestion progresses to the more easily recognized pattern of pulmonary oedema. Later developments may be the appearance of dilated lymphatics at the costo-phrenic angles (Kerley lines) and of pleural effusions, but these imply oedema of at least several days' duration.

Accurate measurement of pulmonary venous pressure is indicated only when some of the more drastic forms of treatment of left ventricular failure have to be used (see below). Conventional cardiac catheterization was not free from risk in patients with recent ischaemia, but the recent development of the Swan—Ganz catheter has permitted measurement of pulmonary artery and pulmonary vein ('wedge') pressures, and the collection of pulmonary artery blood samples as safe bedside procedures. The fine catheter has a double lumen, one of which is used to fill a small balloon at the tip with carbon dioxide or air. Once the tip of the catheter is within the thorax, the balloon is inflated; by moving within the blood-stream it guides the catheter rapidly through the right heart to the pulmonary artery (see Fig. 1.14). Fluoroscopy is helpful but not essential.

Because some degree of left ventricular dysfunction occurs in all patients with myocardial infarction, it is our practice to give a mild diuretic as a precautionary measure over the first few days in all uncomplicated cases. There is no evidence that this forestalls later problems, but no harm will result provided the drug is discontinued several days before any pre-discharge assessment is made. In the presence of tachycardia, triple rhythm, marked cardiomegaly, or definite pulmonary congestion, frusemide 40 mg b.d., together with potassium supplements should be used. The diuretic regime can be reduced or perhaps discontinued if the subsequent course is favourable. The more potent diuretics are also used in the presence of congestive (right-sided) failure, but a venous pressure up to 6 cm may be acceptable, particularly in the early hours after inferior infarction, or in the presence of a low output state which would be exacerbated by hypovolaemia. Digoxin should be used only if tachycardia or other evidence of failure persist despite treatment with diuretics, for cardiac glycosides may enhance the risk of ventricular arrhythmias. If digoxin is used, it must be remembered that the drug is excreted via the urinary tract, and

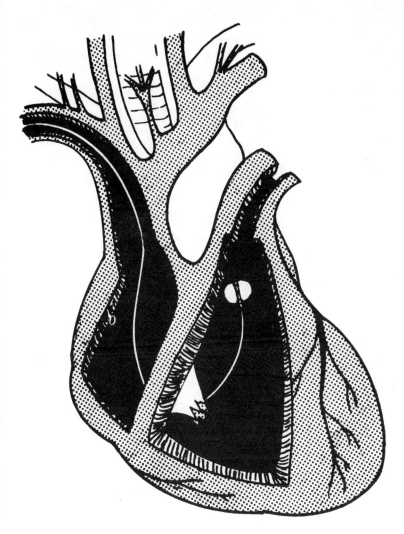

Fig. 1.14. Illustration of Swan—Ganz catheter being 'floated' through the right ventricle towards the pulmonary artery. The inflated balloon at the tip is readily carried forward in the blood stream. (Reproduced from Edwards Laboratories leaflet with permission of Genito-Urinary Mfg. Co. Ltd.)

maintenance doses must be reduced in the presence of impaired renal function.

The treatment of pulmonary oedema is a 'medical emergency' for even if the patient is not unduly distressed his condition is precarious. Treatment should be as follows:

i. Diamorphine (5 mg) or morphine (10 mg) by slow intravenous injection unless these or similar drugs have recently been used for the relief of pain. They act by reducing venous return, and thereby help to restore the balance between the output of right and left ventricles.

ii. Oxygen, preferably by a mask, with a reservoir bag to permit a high concentration.

iii. In severe cases, sphygmomanometer cuffs can be inflated around the thighs to 60 mm Hg, further to reduce venous return and act as a 'bloodless venesection'. They should not be left inflated for more than 30 minutes. By inducing venous stasis they may well encourage the formation of thrombi in the lower limbs.

iv. In severe or moderately severe cases, aminophylline 250 to 375 mg by slow intravenous injection over at least 10 minutes. This may favourably influence both airways' resistance and myocardial contractility.

v. Digoxin in 0·5 mg doses by intravenous infusion. This is most conveniently achieved by diluting the digoxin in 5% dextrose and administering by drip. Rapid digitalization has dangers, but a reasonable compromise is to give the first dose over 30 minutes, the second over 60 minutes, and a third and final dose over 120 minutes.

vi. Diuretics probably do not influence the early course of acute pulmonary oedema, but 20 mg frusemide should be given intravenously to reduce the risk of recurrence. Oral maintenance treatment can be initiated simultaneously.

Acute pulmonary oedema may be precipitated by the injudicious use of β-adrenergic blocking agents in patients with seriously impaired left ventricular function. In such cases, digoxin, aminophylline, and glucagon (50 μg/kg body weight intravenously over 3 minutes) will help to restore myocardial contractility.

Occasionally pulmonary oedema may prove persistent and

refractory to conventional treatment. The prognosis in such cases is poor, but some patients do eventually make a reasonable recovery if they can be tided over the early phase of their illness. More aggressive forms of treatment may be particularly justifiable if deterioration has been caused by a complication potentially remediable by subsequent surgery. Some of the less frequently used measures are as follows:

i. Isoprenaline infusion, in a dose 1 to 4 μg per minute by constant rate infusion pump or carefully controlled drip. This must not be regarded as 'conventional' treatment because it increases myocardial oxygen requirements and may actually extend the size of the infarct. It may also increase susceptibility to arrhythmias. Before the infusion is started, the following haemodynamic measurements should be made if circumstances permit: arterial pressure, mixed venous saturation, and pulmonary artery 'wedge' pressure. The initial dose is 1 μg per minute, and this can be increased progressively provided a favourable haemodynamic response is obtained, and provided an excessive tachycardia does not occur. If isoprenaline is prescribed without regard to the response, a heavy metabolic price may be paid by the failing heart, with no favourable effect obtained in return.

ii. Peritoneal dialysis. Pulmonary oedema can be cleared fairly rapidly by the use of hypertonic solutions, but excessive hypovolaemia may cause critically low output states.

iii. Intra-aortic balloon counter-pulsation. Devices for counter-pulsation are commercially available, and used widely in the United States. A long balloon or series of balloons are positioned high in the thoracic aorta and inflated rapidly with helium each diastole (Fig. 1.15). The balloon is deflated immediately before systole. The left ventricle therefore pumps against an artificially low pressure, yet has the benefit of an augmented coronary artery filling pressure during diastole.

iv. Artificial ventilation. Although arterial oxygen saturation may be increased, cardiac output following myocardial infarction is usually reduced by positive pressure ventilation and the patient's general condition is rarely improved. However, a patient with refractory failure who is profoundly distressed by dyspnoea can be relieved by the use of large doses of opiates if ventilation is supported.

47

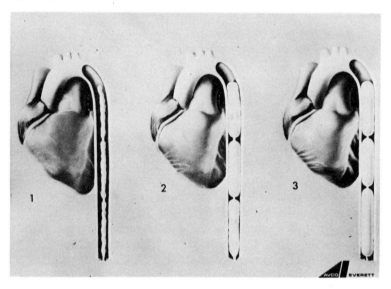

Fig. 1.15. A diagrammatic representation of the Avco intra-aortic balloon pump in-situ. The balloon is inflated rapidly each diastole, providing a further 'boost' to the circulation. It is deflated immediately before systole, thus abruptly reducing arterial pressure and the work of the heart. (Reproduced with permission of Kontron Instruments Ltd.)

Cardiogenic Shock

Cardiogenic shock represents a severe degree of 'forward' heart failure in which cardiac output is critically impaired despite an adequate venous return. It is manifested by pallor, hypotension (systolic pressure less than 90 mm Hg), sweating, oliguria, and frequently by altered consciousness.

Enhanced sympathetic tone acting on the capacitance vessels usually prevents venous 'pooling' and ensures an increased right atrial filling pressure. Because coronary artery disease impairs left ventricular function more than right ventricular function, cardiogenic shock is generally accompanied by pulmonary congestion or pulmonary oedema. The patient should lie in the position he finds most comfortable. Nothing is gained by encouraging him to lie flat. The following measures must be taken when appropriate:

i. The relief of pain. This has first priority not only for the general well-being of the patient but also because pain intensifies shock and increases susceptibility to arrhythmias. Diamorphine is the most effective analgesic, and should be given by slow intravenous injection (p. 13).

ii. The correction of any arrhythmias (p. 41). In the presence of cardiogenic shock, tachyarrhythmias should usually be treated by DC shock, both to achieve a quick response and also to avoid as far as possible the use of suppressant drugs which impair myocardial contractility.

iii. The correction of metabolic acidosis by measured amounts of sodium bicarbonate. Acidosis may result from inadequate perfusion of tissue. It increases susceptibility to arrhythmias and further lowers cardiac output by reducing the contractile power of the ventricles.

iv. Oxygen therapy. Marked lowering of the pO_2 is almost invariable in cardiogenic shock. This is due both to pulmonary congestion and also to ventilation-perfusion imbalance. Unfortunately, the hypoxia cannot be corrected fully by oxygen therapy, but a worthwhile improvement is usually achieved especially when high inspiratory concentrations are attained by using large flow rates of humidified oxygen and a mask with a reservoir bag. Some conscious patients will not tolerate a mask and in them nasal tubes may make a small contribution.

v. Digitalization. Digoxin should be administered as in other forms of heart failure. Slow intravenous infusion (p. 46) is appropriate, but the dose must be controlled with care because patients with cardiogenic shock are particularly prone to arrhythmias. The drug should be discontinued if the patient's progress suggests that failure can be controlled without it. Diuretics are used according to the usual indications.

If cardiogenic shock remains severe after the relief of pain and the correction of arrhythmias and acidosis, the prognosis is very poor with an expected mortality exceeding 80 per cent. Other measures must be taken which demand careful control. After suitable sedation, a catheter should be positioned in the superior vena cava, and if practicable a Swan—Ganz catheter (p. 44) should be floated into a distal pulmonary artery. The following measurements can then be made:

right atrial pressure
indirect left atrial pressure
mixed venous saturation
arterial pressure (by sphymomanometer)

A careful check must be kept of urinary output but preferably without catheterization. Arterial pH must be checked as frequently as necessary to combat any tendency to persistent acidosis.

At this stage further treatment depends upon the pressure readings from the venous catheters. On rare occasions, serious hypotension occurs in patients with myocardial infarction with a near-normal or even low right atrial pressure and a left atrial pressure less than 15 mm Hg. This implies a failure of the reflexes which usually ensure an adequate venous return, with relative hypovolaemia complicating or even replacing true cardiogenic shock. The syndrome thus resembles hypovolaemic shock, but although it is treated in a similar manner, the effects of volume expansion must be monitored carefully. It is prudent to start treatment with a rapid infusion of 500 ml 5% dextrose. If a favourable response is obtained on cardiac output (reflected by mixed venous saturation) and on arterial pressure, *without a dangerous increment in left atrial pressure*, the dextrose is followed by an infusion of plasma expander such as dextran, or — if large volumes are needed — by blood. If no favourable response is obtained as a result of the dextrose infusion, or if left atrial pressure rises markedly, no lasting harm will result because the dextrose is quickly dissipated throughout the whole fluid compartment.

The syndrome of true cardiogenic shock is very much more common, and in these instances the right atrial pressure will be more than 10 cm water (i.e. 7·5 mm Hg) above the sternal angle. Even if left atrial pressure cannot be monitored, a fairly reliable rule-of-thumb suggests that it will be at least twice as high as right atrial pressure. Treatment by volume expansion is therefore contraindicated and if attempted may precipitate pulmonary oedema. An attempt should be made to increase cardiac output with an inotropic agent and at the present time isoprenaline is regarded as the drug of choice. The initial dose should be 1 μg per minute, regulated by a constant infusion pump. This can be increased progressively to 4 or 5 μg per minute provided each increment is matched by a favourable haemodynamic response and provided an excessive tachycardia does not occur.

If isoprenaline is contraindicated because of tachycardia (heart rate more than 120 per minute), recurrent arrhythmias, or because of the recent use of β-blocking drugs, glucagon may be used instead in a dose of 0·05 mg per kg by slow intravenous injection over 2 or 3 minutes. This may be repeated hourly, if necessary, but blood sugar must be carefully monitored to avoid hyperglycaemia or hypoglycaemia. Adrenaline, noradrenaline, and similar synthetic sympathomimetics may increase blood pressure by an α-stimulating effect, but in patients with cardiogenic shock cardiac output is rarely increased by these measures. A physician must remember that a heavy metabolic price is paid by the heart for treatment with catecholamines and they must never be used if a commensurate 'return' is not achieved.

Myocardial assist devices (p. 47) are effective in the short term for the treatment of cardiogenic shock, but if simpler methods fail it is very unlikely that enough viable left ventricular muscle remains to support any useful life.

Pericarditis

Pericarditis occurs very commonly after transmural myocardial infarction as a result of direct involvement of the visceral pericardium. The most frequent clinical manifestation is pain. The pain is similar in character to that of ischaemic heart pain, but it tends to radiate less and it is *exacerbated by inspiration.* Patients may obtain relief by changes in posture, for example by leaning forwards. Pericardial pain usually occurs 24 to 48 hours after the infarct, sometimes before the original discomfort has abated. Any patient who suffers persistent pain or recurrent pain should be questioned about the relationship to breathing and posture, for otherwise the presence of the complication may be unrecognized. Less common manifestations which may occur if the pericarditis is widespread include fever which may be more severe and more prolonged than that usually associated with infarction, and supraventricular arrhythmias especially atrial fibrillation. Thus, *p*ericarditis causes *p*ain, *p*rolonged *p*yrexia, and *p*alpitation. A friction rub may be heard, but it is often transient, and its absence in no way negates the diagnosis.

The complication is usually benign, though tamponade may occur as a result of intrapericardial bleeding, particularly if the patient is anticoagulated. A temporary reduction in the dose of heparin or oral anticoagulants is therefore indicated if pericarditis is diagnosed. Indomethacin is remarkably effective as an analgesic for pericardial pain, but drug interaction due to competition for protein binding sites must be remembered if the patient is receiving treatment with oral anticoagulants.

The post-infarction syndrome (Dressler's syndrome) is a second cause of pericarditis following myocardial infarction. This may present 7 to 21 days after the infarct with recurrence of fever, pericardial or pleural pain with or without effusions, tachycardia, heart failure, and a very high ESR. It is thought to have an auto-immune basis. Differential diagnoses which must often be considered include further myocardial infarction, infection (especially from intravenous canulae), and pulmonary emboli. The syndrome is usually self-limiting. It is treated symptomatically with analgesics and, if necessary, with diuretics. If the symptoms are very troublesome or very prolonged the condition may be suppressed by steroids.

Pulmonary Emboli

Patients with myocardial infarction are at special risk from pulmonary emboli: they are kept at rest in bed, movement may be reduced by heavy sedation, and venous stasis is promoted if resting cardiac output is reduced. The sensitive ^{131}I fibrinogen test has revealed thrombus formation in the leg veins of up to 40 per cent of patients who are seriously ill after coronary attacks. In the past, about 5 per cent of all deaths from myocardial infarction were due to pulmonary emboli, but the proportion fell with the introduction of anticoagulants and the tendency towards more rapid mobilization. Our own policy is to allow 6 days of bed-rest for patients with uncomplicated infarcts if they are anticoagulated (see p. 12), and 3 if they are not. The very elderly are kept in bed only for the duration of pain or hypotension.

Systemic Emboli

Clot commonly forms on the damaged endocardium underlying an infarct, and in some cases may occupy as much as a quarter of the left ventricular cavity. If clot breaks loose it may embolize to brain, kidney, mesenteric artery, spleen, or limb. Cerebral emboli may cause permanent and tragic disability: no effective treatment is available. Large emboli affecting the limbs can be removed surgically, but in the presence of a recent infarct local anaesthesia with adequate sedation is preferable to general anaesthesia. Anticoagulants probably reduce the incidence of systemic emboli, but little firm evidence is available on this point.

Ventricular Aneurysm

In some patients with transmural infarction the area of necrosed myocardium is replaced by thin fibrous tissue which bulges out-wards during ventricular systole, and may gradually enlarge to form an aneurysmal sac. Such dyskinetic areas occur most commonly in the distribution of the anterior descending coronary artery. Although ventricular aneurysms may grow to an impressive size they do not rupture. They are usually lined by laminated and organizing blood clot, the inner layers of which may remain friable for many months. The risks to the patient are three-fold; from systemic emboli, from left ventricular failure, and from arrhythmias. Left ventricular failure occurs not only because of a reduction in the area of contractile myocardium but also because much of the energy of contraction is wasted in expanding the aneurysmal sac, a situation haemodynamically analogous to that in mitral regurgitation.

The diagnosis may often be suspected if palpation of the praecordium suggests an expansile systolic impulse. It is supported electrocardiographically by persistent ST elevation (of more than 6 weeks' duration) in leads showing pathological monophasic Q waves, and radiologically by a characteristic bulge along the left border of the cardiac silhouette. The most reliable investigation to confirm an aneurysm is left ventricular angiography, for simple screening of the heart may fail to detect paradoxical movement, especially on the inferior surface of the ventricle.

53

The frequency of embolic complications can probably be reduced by long-term anticoagulants. Failure and arrhythmias can usually be controlled by conventional methods, but in refractory cases resection of the aneurysm may be indicated and is sometimes dramatically successful. Cardiac catheterization and angiography should therefore be considered in patients with left ventricular failure which does not respond to adequate drug therapy and which persists for two to three months after infarction.

Papillary Muscle Dysfunction

Effective closure of the mitral valve depends upon the integrity of the whole mitral apparatus: valves, chordae, and papillary muscles. When the left ventricle contracts, the papillary muscles also shorten and enable the chordae to hold the free edges of the valve in apposition, resisting the pressure within the ventricular cavity.

If the papillary muscles are involved in the ischaemic process they may not contract effectively: this failure of function allows the edges of the mitral valve to prolapse into the left atrium and so gives rise to mitral regurgitation. An opposite effect can occur as a result of chronic dilation of the left ventricle: the combined length of chordae plus papillary muscles may be insufficient to permit full closure of the mitral valve, and this, too, causes regurgitation.

The murmur of mitral regurgitation due to papillary muscle dysfunction may resemble the murmur of rheumatic mitral incompetence or may differ from it in several respects: the timing may be late-systolic, the radiation may be towards the base of the heart, and it sometimes varies with posture. In most cases papillary muscle dysfunction is a relatively unimportant incidental finding, but it can be a contributory cause of left ventricular failure.

A papillary muscle may become necrosed because of total occlusion of its arterial supply, in which case it is likely to rupture under the strain transmitted by the chordae. This causes severe mitral regurgitation of sudden onset which is liable to be followed by acute pulmonary oedema. The differential diagnosis of an abrupt onset of left ventricular failure

54

following an infarct, accompanied by a loud systolic murmur, lies between papillary muscle rupture and rupture of the ventricular septum. In either event the failure usually proves refractory to conventional medical therapy. Urgent investigation by left ventricular angiography is indicated in suitable cases with a view to replacement of the mitral valve or repair of the septal defect. Unfortunately, the operative risks of both procedures are high, but the late results may be satisfactory in those who survive surgery.

Rupture of the Heart

Rupture may involve the intraventricular septum, and a large left-to-right shunt then occurs through the acquired septal defect. Severe pulmonary oedema follows. The septum has a rich blood supply, and this complication is unlikely to supervene unless both the anteroseptal and inferior aspects of the myocardium are infarcted. The murmur is typically pansystolic and parasternal. Cardiac catheterization and the confirmation of a shunt differentiates ruptured septum from rupture of a papillary muscle. Surgical treatment is an urgent necessity (see above).

Rupture of the free wall of the left ventricle causes immediate tamponade. This is manifest by sudden collapse usually accompanied by severe bradycardia. Death occurs within minutes. There is no effective treatment.

CONVALESCENCE

The responsibility of the physician does not end with the supervision of the acute stages of a coronary attack and the treatment of complications. One of his most important tasks is to prepare the patient for effective rehabilitation. Clear advice must be offered for a period of increasing activity. Walking is the safest exercise. Sudden strenuous exertion should be discouraged, especially when accompanied by emotional stress (missing a bus is preferable to ventricular fibrillation!). The patient must aim to be fitter after his convalescence than before his attack, and to return as far as possible to a normal life. Unfortunately, cardiac neurosis is common, and many survivors of coronary attacks never return to work despite their making an excellent recovery. This represents a failure of treatment for which the physician bears a heavy burden of responsibility.

Chapter 2

Respiratory Failure

G. GERSON

CAUSES OF RESPIRATORY FAILURE

ENDOTRACHEAL INTUBATION
   Complications

TRACHEOSTOMY
   Technique
   Complications

OXYGEN THERAPY
   Indications
   Methods of Administration

HUMIDIFICATION

PHYSIOTHERAPY

ARTIFICIAL VENTILATION
   Indications
   Initiation
   Regulation
   Termination and Weaning
   Types of Ventilator
   Complications of Mechanical Ventilation

57

The successful management of acute respiratory failure by supportive intermittent positive pressure ventilation was probably the foremost single factor responsible for the development of Intensive Care Units. Both the prevention and treatment of respiratory insufficiency have taken rapid strides forward with the advent of this therapy and with improvements and refinements in the techniques being used, there has been an associated reduction in mortality.

In this chapter the general principles governing the management of acute respiratory failure will be considered, since these principles are common to all cases regardless of the particular cause of the respiratory inadequacy.

CAUSES OF RESPIRATORY FAILURE

Respiratory failure occurs where pulmonary gas exchange is so disturbed as to lead to hypoxaemia with or without hypercapnia.

Derangement of respiratory function may be due to many factors acting either primarily on the lungs by a central or peripheral mechanism, or secondarily on the lungs following disturbances in function of other organ systems.

1. Conditions directly affecting the lungs.
2. Conditions affecting the respiratory muscles or their neural control.
3. Traumatic conditions directly affecting the mechanical act of breathing.
4. Conditions involving other organ systems and secondarily resulting in respiratory disturbances.

1. Conditions Directly Affecting the Lungs

(a) *Acute Infections.* Pulmonary infections leading to respiratory failure are seen in the debilitated and old, and in those suffering from chronic pulmonary disease. In winter and at times of influenza epidemics previously healthy and young individuals may develop pulmonary infections severe enough to require admission to Intensive Care Units. Increasing hypoxaemia and dyspnoea followed by exhaustion may necessitate the use of artificial ventilation. Acute infections may be superimposed on chronic respiratory disease or on long standing respiratory muscle weakness.

(b) *Bronchial Asthma.* This condition affects all age groups. An attack may be triggered off by an acute infection. Where severe bronchospasm and constriction occur, intensive therapy may be required.

(c) *Pneumothorax.* This may occur following rupture of an emphysematous bulla, trauma to the chest wall leading to fractured ribs which lacerate the pleura and underlying lung, or after the introduction of a needle through the chest wall. In patients who are in an Intensive Care Unit, pneumothorax may follow attempts at subclavian vein cannulation. A tension pneumothorax may occur where, due to a valvular action of the visceral pleura, air enters but cannot leave the pleural cavity. The affected lung collapses and the tension of the air in the pleural space pushes the mediastinum to the opposite side compressing the opposite lung. Great respiratory distress may result, requiring immediate relief.

(d) *Trauma to the Lungs.* This is frequently associated with injuries to the chest wall following road traffic accidents or industrial injuries or falls from heights. Contusion and bleeding into lung tissues may result in interference with aeration of large areas of lung.

2. Conditions Affecting the Respiratory Muscles or their Neural Control

(a) *Head Injuries.* Accidents or surgery may damage the respiratory centre directly, or cause haemorrhage or oedema and a rise in intracranial pressure. The latter may result in respiratory centre involvement.

(b) *Cerebro-Vascular Accidents.* Similarly these conditions cause a rise in intracranial pressure and respiratory centre compression.

(c) *Agents used in Anaesthesia.* General anaesthetics and analgesics may depress the respiratory centre sufficiently to cause or contribute towards respiratory failure. Muscle relaxants act on the neuromuscular junction, and their action is to paralyze voluntary musculature. Artificial ventilation is used throughout their duration of action, but their action may be prolonged under certain conditions especially in association with electrolyte disturbances. Certain drugs such as streptomycin and neomycin may prolong the activity of muscle relaxants.

(d) *Guillain–Barré Syndrome.* This condition is an acute infective polyneuritis, characterized by bilateral peripheral muscle weakness, difficulty in respiration and sometimes swallowing, together with some loss of sensation.

(e) *Tetanus.* Spasms, inadequate ventilation and sometimes aspiration of gastric contents may all lead to respiratory failure.

(f) *Poliomyelitis.* With the introduction of vaccine, this disease is rarely seen.

(g) *Poisonings.* Barbiturates form the commonest group of drugs responsible for respiratory failure due to central depression. Glutethimide overdosage can also cause respiratory failure.

Analgesics such as morphine, heroin, papaveretum, pethidine, phenoperidine and fentanyl when used injudiciously may cause respiratory failure. This may be seen where they are repeated too soon by the intramuscular route in patients who are shocked. In such cases the initial dose has not had time to work owing to the poor circulation. A relative overdosage may be seen in the post-operative period where other factors may augment respiratory depression.

Any tranquilizer or sedative taken in sufficient excess may cause respiratory depression, and this applies even to those drugs which are often claimed to be harmless in this respect. When alcohol is taken in addition, these effects will be enhanced.

Aspirin overdosage does not usually result in respiratory failure.

Carbon monoxide, a constituent of coal gas, causes anoxia because of its affinity for haemoglobin which is much greater than that of oxygen. This form of poisoning is becoming less common with the introduction of carbon monoxide-free natural gas from the North Sea.

(h) *Myasthenia Gravis.* Respiratory failure may occur as a result of progression of the disease, or following excessive administration of anti-cholinesterases in an attempt to control the symptoms, since such an excess may itself cause respiratory depression.

Respiratory failure is also seen following thymectomy which is used as a treatment for this condition, or following major abdominal or thoracic surgery in affected patients.

(i) *Muscular Dystrophies.* Various conditions of muscular weakness may give rise to respiratory inadequacy.

(j) *High Spinal Cord Injuries.* These will result in respiratory depression due to the respiratory muscle weakness following the nerve injury.

3. Conditions Affecting the Mechanical Act of Breathing

(a) *Crushed Chest.* Chest wall injuries may give rise to fractures of the sternum and ribs. A flail chest may result, in which paradoxical movement of the unstable chest wall occurs on breathing. As a result pulmonary gas exchange rapidly becomes inadequate.

(b) *Surgery.* Many factors are involved in the development of post-operative respiratory failure. Interference with lung expansion by pain is common, especially after thoracic and upper abdominal incisions. Obesity and the magnitude of the surgery are contributory factors.

Pre-existing lung disease and debility may of course be superimposed on the mechanical limitations.

4. Conditions Involving Other Organ Systems and Secondarily Resulting in Respiratory Disturbances

(a) *Cardiovascular System*
  (i) Myocardial infarction is followed by arterial hypoxaemia probably due to alteration in ventilation perfusion ratios.

(ii) Haemorrhage and pulmonary emboli interfere with normal perfusion of the lungs. This results in an increased physiological dead space with inadequate oxygenation of the arterial blood and inadequate elimination of carbon-dioxide.

(b) *Septicaemia.* In this condition micro-embolization of infected material to the pulmonary vessels may contribute to pulmonary dysfunction.

(c) *Multi-system Failure.* Exhaustion and general debility are frequently associated with respiratory failure. Patients with failure of more than one system should be carefully observed for the earliest evidence of deterioration of respiratory function.

ENDOTRACHEAL INTUBATION

This is indicated where the patient is:
1. Unable to maintain his airway by other means.
2. Needs artificial ventilation.
3. Requires aspiration of the respiratory tract, or
4. To prevent inhalation of foreign material such as vomit or blood in the mouth or pharynx.

Endotracheal tubes are made of rubber or plastic. The latter are less irritant to the larynx and trachea and are therefore more suitable for use in Intensive Care Units, where they may have to stay in place for days rather than hours. (See Fig. 2.1.)

Tubes with inflatable cuffs are used in order that:

1. Gastric contents and other foreign matter may be prevented from contaminating the respiratory tract, and
2. So that if the patient receives artificial ventilation there will be no gas leak around the tube and precise volumes of inspired air and oxygen can be delivered and confirmed.

Endotracheal tubes may be inserted through the nose or mouth. The diameter of the tube inserted is limited in the former case by that of the nasal passage. A muscle relaxant such as suxamethonium given after the patient is anaesthetized may be used to facilitate introduction of the tube. Many patients who require intubation in the Intensive Care Unit, will not be able to

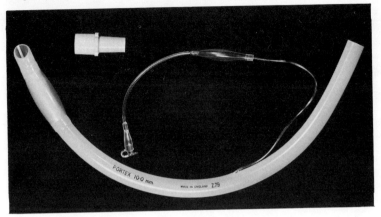

Fig. 2.1. Plastic endotracheal tube with connection.

tolerate a general anaesthetic and will need only some topical anaesthesia to the pharynx, larynx and trachea applied through the mouth or by transtracheal injection through the cricothyroid membrane. A laryngoscope is used to identify the vocal cords and so introduce the tube.

The endotracheal tube is carefully fixed in position around the mouth so that it will not move up or down the trachea. Both lung apices are auscultated to ensure that the right bronchus has not been intubated.

From the time of insertion of the tube, all inspired gases must be humidified, since the tube bypasses the normal humidifying mechanisms of the nasopharynx.

Complications

(a) *Vocal cord damage.* This is usually transitory provided that the tube is not left in place too long. Prolonged intubation causes ulceration which can lead to fibrosis and narrowing.

(b) *Tracheal damage.* This is chiefly stenosis at the level of the inflatable cuff (see tracheostomy complications) but is seldom seen following intubation of only two or three days.

TRACHEOSTOMY

When a tube has to be kept in the trachea for more than 4—5 days in adults, whether for artificial ventilation or maintenance of an airway, tracheostomy is usually considered. Factors which will tend to influence the decision towards performing a tracheostomy are, anticipated artificial ventilation for a long period, and inability to tolerate oral or nasal endotracheal tube without heavy sedation. Factors mitigating against tracheostomy are, acute on chronic chest pathology in patients who may develop recurrent acute chest infections, and patients with coagulation defects.

The operation is performed with an oral or nasal endotracheal tube in position, so that control of the airway is maintained until the tracheostomy tube is inserted through the incision. Only rarely is it not possible to have an endotracheal tube in situ prior to the operation.

Technique

Anaesthesia:
  Inhalational anaesthetics or intravenous agents may be used. The presence of an endotracheal tube by safeguarding the airway, allows the operation to be unhurried. A variety of agents and techniques can be used dependant on the physical condition of the patient. In general the greater the degree of cardiovascular depression, the less anaesthetic agent the patient will require. The respirations may need to be artificially supported. In exceptional circumstances where an endotracheal tube cannot be passed, the operation may be performed under a local anaesthetic.

Operation: A transverse skin incision is made over the second and third tracheal cartilages about 1 inch below the cricoid cartilage. Using blunt midline dissection and a pair of small Langenbecks retractors held by an assistant, all planes are retracted laterally in turn until the trachea is exposed. A ∩ shaped flap is cut in the trachea large enough to insert the tracheostomy tube.

  32–36 French gauge for females.
  36–40 French gauge for males.

The flap of cartilage is sewn down to the lower edge of the incision and the tracheostomy tube is inserted, withdrawing the endotracheal tube at the same time, but not through the vocal cords. If there is difficulty in inserting the tracheostomy tube, the endotracheal tube can then be easily replaced.

The skin is closed with sutures and the tube is held in place by tapes, which are tied round the side of the neck in a bow. A Melolin non-adherent dressing is placed over the incision under the flanges of the tracheostomy tube.

Types of Tube

For mechanical ventilation a cuffed tracheostomy tube is needed and a plastic tube such as the Portex one is generally used. Metal, red rubber and reinforced latex tubes are also available. Portex plastic tubes are implantation tested in rabbits to ensure that they consist of non-toxic material. They are gamma-irradiated to sterilize them. The cuffs should be pre-stretched prior to use (see complications). During the first 24 hours following a tracheostomy there may be difficulty in replacing the tube should it come out or be misplaced before a track has formed. Tracheal dilators, laryngoscope and endotracheal tube must be readily available during this period.

Care of Tracheostomy

Adequate humidification should be provided through the tracheostomy tube from the time of insertion. Aspiration of secretions should be performed as necessary and samples sent to the laboratory for culture and sensitivity regularly.

Suction through the tracheostomy tube is performed by a catheter under sterile conditions. Suction should be preceded by ample oxygenation and should not continue for longer than 15 seconds. Cardiac arrest may occur in hypoxaemic patients who are suctioned for too long. The cuff should be inflated if ventilation is necessary or if there is any danger of inhalation. The cuff may be released at intervals though it is not certain that this reduces the risk of tracheal stenosis. The tube is changed if the cuff leaks or any obstruction occurs.

Complications

1. *Disconnection between the ventilator and the tracheostomy tube.* This is particularly dangerous in patients who have been

given muscle relaxants in order to facilitate the control of artificial ventilation. Correctly fitting connections and apnoea monitors help to diminish this risk.

2. *Misplacement.* The tube may be inserted into pre-tracheal tissues or may be too long and enter the right bronchus. In the latter case air entry will be impaired on auscultation of the left lung.

3. *Blockage of secretions.* Efficient humidification should help to avert most of these problems which are due to incrustation of the tube by viscid secretions.

4. *Ulceration.* The walls of the trachea may be eroded by the tube or cuff, leading to perforation or erosion of an artery. This is commoner with metal tubes.

5. *The incision may become infected.* Ps. pyocyaneus is a commensal commonly found in the stoma of a tracheostomy and needs no treatment in the absence of signs of active respiratory tract infection (pyrexia, raised WBC, pneumonia).

6. *Surgical emphysema.* This is seen especially when the incision is tightly sewn up.

7. *Stenosis.* This usually occurs within the first months after extubation, and is most commonly found at the level at which the cuff was inflated. Ulceration at this level is followed by fibrotic stenosis. Prevention of this condition which is due to pressure necrosis may be aided by pre-stretching the cuffs of the tracheostomy tubes with 25 ml of air whilst the tube is immersed in hot water. This enables the cuffs to be inflated to the usual degree using a lower inflating pressure. New cuffs are at present being developed which possess a large volume at a low inflation pressure. Treatment of the established condition is by resection and anastomosis of the trachea.

OXYGEN THERAPY

Oxygen plays a vital role in the prophylaxis of incipient respiratory failure and the management of the established condition.

Since intracellular metabolism depends upon oxidative processes, a failure of the respiratory system to transfer adequate supplies of oxygen from the inspired air to the blood and so to the cells will result in a depression of aerobic metabolism within the cell, and ultimately in cell necrosis. Vital organs such as the brain and heart are highly susceptible to a diminution of their oxygen supplies.

Hypoxaemia is commonly found in patients in the Intensive Care Unit, and compensatory mechanisms such as hyperventilation and increased catecholamine release may help to correct the deficiencies in arterial blood oxygen content. Unfortunately, patients in Intensive Care Units are frequently anaemic (haemorrhage and chronic anaemic states) and many patients have lowered cardiac outputs, so that compensatory mechanisms to improve circulatory transport of oxygen may not be available. In these circumstances, a relatively moderate fall of arterial oxygen tension may result in harmful effects. Whilst adding oxygen to inspired air may only improve haemoglobin saturation slightly, it will increase the oxygen in solution in the plasma which can provide an appreciable additional source of oxygen for the tissues, when considered in relation to the total amount of oxygen uptake by the tissues from the blood. Hyperbaric oxygen will increase this fraction of the blood oxygen even further, so that sufficient may be carried in solution to meet the whole of the body's requirements. These factors assume increased importance in the presence of circulatory failure with a lowered haemoglobin as occurs following a large haemorrhage. Oxygen is given in these conditions of shock even in the absence of any lung impairment, so that an increase of oxygen in solution in the plasma will help to compensate for the deficiencies in oxygen transport mechanisms within the cardiovascular system.

The management of hypoxaemia in the first instance will, in addition to adequate oxygen administration, include attention to the aetiological factors concerned, such as:

1. Cardiac failure therapy: digitalis and diuretics..
2. Humidification and physiotherapy with postural drainage.
3. Tracheo-bronchial toilet.
4. Bronchodilators.
5. Chest aspiration.
6. Antibiotics.
7. Steroids.

Indications for Oxygen Therapy in Intensive Care Units

1. *Lowered PO$_2$*. Apart from obvious acute pulmonary infection which is the commonest cause, this may occur in a variety of conditions met with in the Intensive Care Unit, including those patients who are unconscious from overdosage of drugs, post-operative patients and almost any severely debilitated patient. The association of hypoxaemia and the post-operative state (upper abdominal and thoracic surgery in particular) is well recognized. It is important that the absence of cyanosis is not relied upon as an indication for withholding additional oxygen, since its presence is dependent on haemoglobin level and blood flow, and its recognition is also subject to observer error. When present it is certainly an indication for giving oxygen. Sufficient oxygen should be given to restore the PO$_2$ to a level above 80 mm Hg, taking into account the age and normal level of PO$_2$ in those patients who have been suffering from long standing pulmonary disease. It is difficult to be precise in correcting oxygenation in patients who are breathing spontaneously, but if there is any doubt as to their cardiovascular status it is safest to aim at higher PO$_2$'s whilst trying to avoid a PO$_2$ of above 150 mm Hg (see pulmonary oxygen toxicity). Following cardiac arrest or in severe emergencies should be given 100% oxygen until the immediate danger is over. Measurement of arterial PO$_2$'s is performed as often as necessary to maintain them at the desired level.

2. *Patients with Lowered Cardiac Outputs.* This includes patients who are shocked due to haemorrhage or have suffered recent heart damage such as myocardial infarction, or undergone open-heart surgery.

3. *Chronic Lung Disease.* A special indication for restriction of the percentage of oxygen given to a patient, is in those patients who suffer from chronic lung disease with a raised PCO$_2$ to which they have become tolerant. These patients depend on a hypoxic drive and if this is withdrawn by provision of too much oxygen, they may develop a state of CO$_2$ narcosis. Such patients are occasionally met with in Intensive Care Units in an acute exacerbation of their chronic chest condition. The treat-

ment of these patients depends on the principle of giving sufficient oxygen to improve their lowered oxygen saturation without allowing their PCO_2 to rise to dangerous levels.

Methods of Administering Oxygen

Face Masks. There are several patterns of masks available including the MC mask, Pneumask and Harris mask which provide up to 50% oxygen in the inspired air if there is a high flow rate of oxygen. Higher percentages can be achieved by using a mask with a reservoir bag, although this may result in a larger dead space, which could be more dangerous in the event of failure of the oxygen supply. The Ventimask is designed to deliver fixed concentrations of O_2 (24%, 28% and 35%) and is therefore useful where controlled therapy is desired as in chronic pulmonary disease with a permanently raised PCO_2 level. If oxygen is to be delivered for any length of time through any of these devices, it is important to humidify it first.

Nasal Catheters. These can be of use provided that the patient does not breathe through his mouth.

Oxygen Tents. These suffer from the disadvantage of being awkward to nurse the patient in, besides not being very effective from the point of view of oxygenation.

HUMIDIFICATION

Ordinarily the inspired air is saturated with water vapour in its passage over the linings of the nasal, oral and pharyngeal cavities. When this process is disturbed by the use of endotracheal tubes or tracheostomy tubes, atmospheric air is not longer humidified. When dry gases such as oxygen are added, the mucus covering the epithelium of the respiratory tract is soon dried up. As a result, the cilia which move this mucus along are damaged, predisposing to the entry of infection into the lungs as well as the formation of viscid secretions which cannot be removed. Humidification of inspired gases is therefore vital whenever endotracheal or tracheostomy tubes are used, with or without mechanical ventilation. At body temperature 44 mg H_2O/litre of gas must be added to the inspired gas to achieve full saturation.

There are three commonly used methods of humidifying inspired gases.

1. *Use of Condenser Humidifier* (e.g. Garthur Humidifier). This contains a mesh or wire which traps expired water vapour and heat and then transfers the moisture and heat to the inspired air. It may be attached to a tracheostomy tube. Its use pre-supposes an initial adequate state of hydration of the patient. The use of oxygen will tend to dry out the water. Organisms may accumulate in the Condenser which needs to be changed frequently.
2. *Heated water baths* (e.g. Cape and East Humidifiers). These humidifiers are an efficient means of humidifying the inspired gases, which are driven over the surface of the water. This is heated by thermostatically controlled elements to about 55°C, which allows the water vapour to cool to 37°C by the time it reaches the patient.
3. *Nebulization* (e.g. Puritan, Bird, Bennett Cascade, De Vilbiss Ultrasonic). These machines produce fine droplets of 0·5—30 μ diameter in a variety of ways. The droplets should be small enough to prevent settling out on their passage to the lungs. The Ultrasonic nebulizers use high frequency vibrations to produce small droplets. They are very efficient and may therefore be dangerous where water retention already exists.

PHYSIOTHERAPY

The techniques of the physiotherapist are frequently used in the management of patients with respiratory problems in the ICU. The efficacy of these techniques cannot readily be assessed quantitatively but many workers in this field are convinced of the value of chest physiotherapy in the prevention and treatment of pulmonary collapse and infection.

Prophylactically, breathing exercises and assistance in coughing help in expanding the lungs and removing secretions. Therapeutic measures include postural drainage and vibratory and percussive techniques to clear the lungs of secretions. In those patients who have an endotracheal tube or tracheostomy tube in situ, the lungs may be expanded using an Ambu or re-breathing bag and as they are allowed to deflate, the physiotherapist can vibrate the chest wall over areas containing any secretions which are recognized on auscultation. This is especially effective when the patient is in the lateral position with the bad side uppermost. The combination of vibration with deflation of the lung from a fully expanded position can succeed in loosening secretions in that part of the lung, so that they may then be removed by suction.

ARTIFICIAL VENTILATION

From the earliest times, man has understood that artifical ventilation had a part to play in the resuscitation of the dying. With the increasing role of artificial ventilation in modern medicine, and in particular the frequent use of intermittent positive pressure ventilation since the polio epidemic of 1951, this form of treatment has come to be used as a prophylactic and therapeutic adjunct in all manner of conditions.

An increase in our knowledge of clinical respiratory physiology has accompanied our progress in the field of respiratory support. Correct management of patients undergoing artificial ventilation now requires regular biochemical investigations, as well as a knowledge of the many complex disturbances that may not only follow artificial ventilation but may also be associated with the conditions necessitating it.

Indications for Artificial Ventilation

The decision as to when to artificially ventilate a patient often poses difficulty for the junior hospital doctor. Severe respiratory depression is usually obvious and its immediate management provides no problems, but patients with respiratory distress of lesser magnitude, or those whose reserve is so limited that they are in potential danger if left to breathe spontaneously, require more careful evaluation.

In recent years prophylactic artificial ventilation of such patients has become increasingly accepted. Those groups who are electively ventialted are recognized and selected by clinical experience of those conditions which are known to lead to deterioration of pulmonary function sufficient to prove a serious

71

hazard to the patient's life. Awareness of such conditions which lead to progressive pulmonary disturbance therefore assumes great importance, and in many instances will influence the decision one would otherwise make on the grounds of quantitatively measured pulmonary function tests alone. Similar considerations apply where the patient is critically ill from multi-system failure, since artificial ventilation will at least ensure that this aspect of the vital functions is as well protected as possible.

Diffuse atelectasis is the common cause of intra-pulmonary shunting of blood past non-ventilated alveoli and may follow episodes of airway closure. Hypoxaemia results and is often associated with small lung volumes. Where hypoxaemia does not respond to maximal oxygen therapy in patients who have reversible disease, artifical mechanical ventilation is indicated.

Pulmonary function is assessed by frequent observation of clinical signs, and by measurements of certain pulmonary tests. The purpose of these repeated recordings is to detect early changes in the lungs and then prevent their advance by appropriate therapy. If artifical ventilation is started early in these cases the ultimate prognosis in terms of both morbidity and mortality is much better than where wide-spread lung changes have been allowed to occur prior to the commencement of such artificial ventilation.

The common conditions leading to respiratory failure which may require artificial ventilation, have been outlined in the section on aetiology. Certain factors aggravate existing pulmonary insufficiency from any cause and these include:

1. Need for analgesics. Where analgesics have to be given to the post-operative patient whose respiratory status is in doubt, small doses given intravaneously can be titrated against the response, so that the minimal dose necessary to relieve pain may be given.
2. Exhaustion.
3. Obesity.
4. Debility.
5. Shock.
6. Muscle weakness.
7. Previous pulmonary disease and emphysema.
8. Rapid fluid infusion.

Respiratory Failure.

Wherever possible in surgery of the extremely ill or debilitated, the need for post-operative elective ventilation should be anticipated, and undertaken prophylactically to prevent adverse pulmonary changes in the immediate post-operative period.

Recordings by nurses. The following observations are charted regularly by the nurses on the Intensive Care Unit.

1. Pulse rate.
2. Respiratory rate.
3. Blood pressure.
4. Inspired oxygen concentration, i.e. percentage of oxygen in inspired gases.
5. Vital capacity.
6. Tidal volume and minute volume.
7. Presence of respiratory distress.

Specialized Tests of Pulmonary Function.

$\left.\begin{array}{l}PaO_2 \\ PaCO_2\end{array}\right\}$ — Adequacy of blood gas exchange.

$\dfrac{VD}{VT}$ — Measure of CO_2 exchange.

A-aDO$_2$ — Measure of O_2 exchange and sensitive index of pulmonary function in acute pulmonary infections or pulmonary oedema.

The explanation of the above symbols is as follows:

PaO$_2$ — Partial pressure of oxygen in arterial blood.
PaCO$_2$ — Partial pressure of carbon dioxide in arterial blood.
VD — Physiological dead space.
VT — Tidal volume.
A-aDO$_2$ — Difference between alveolar and arterial oxygen levels.

X-ray — These changes are usually later in appearance than changes in the other tests mentioned, and therefore active therapy should not await radiological changes which may be associated with irreversible lung damage.

73

HB &
HCT   — Oxygen Transport in the blood.

The accompanying Table I shows accepted ranges for pulmonary function tests and levels at which therapy is commenced.

Table I — Indications for Respiratory Support

		Acceptable range	Chest physical therapy oxygen, close monitoring	Intubation tracheotomy ventilation
Mechanics	Respiratory rate	12—25	25—35	35
	Vital capacity, ml/kg	70—30	30—15	15
	Inspiratory force cm H_2O	100—50	50—25	25
Oxygenation	A-aDO_2 mm Hg*	50—200	200—350	350
	PaO_2 mm Hg	100—75 (air)	200—70 (on mask O_2)	70 (on mask O_2)
Ventilation	V_D/V_T	0·3—0·4	0·4—0·6	0·6
	$PaCO_2$ mm Hg	35—45	45—60	60†

* After 15 minutes of 100% O_2.
† Except in chronic hypercapnia.
From Pontoppidan, H.: Treatment of respiratory failure in nonthoracic trauma. *J. Trauma* 8 : 938—945. 1968. Reprinted with permission from the *Journal of Trauma*.

Changes in the partial pressure of oxygen in the arterial blood (PaO_2) or differences in the alveolar-arterial oxygen levels after breathing 100% oxygen (A-aDO_2) often give early indications of changes in pulmonary gas exchange due to alveolar collapse or consolidation. 100% oxygen can be delivered to the patient using a non-return valve attached to a mouthpiece with the nose clipped. Whilst low absolute values may not in themselves be a sign of imminent failure of oxygenation of vital organs, changes noticed by frequent observations will show a trend towards deterioration of lung function which could be arrested by artificial ventilation before decompensation occurs. Because of compensatory hyperventilation and faster rates of CO_2 diffusion, increases in the arterial carbon dioxide partial pressures usually occur later than falls in arterial oxygen values.

Increase in the ratio of physiological dead space to tidal volume $\left(\dfrac{VD}{VT}\right)$ represents an increase in the amount of alveolar ventilation which is not taking part in gas exchange due to inadequate perfusion of the affected alveoli. When the ratio is above 0·5 ventilation is no longer able to provide satisfactory oxygenation.

Two most easily detected and therefore important indices of the necessity for ventilatory support, are an increasing fall in the PO_2 values of the arterial blood and an increase in the state of exhaustion of the dyspnoeic patient.

The decision to ventilate a patient must also take into consideration his previous pulmonary state and associated ability to live a normal active life, as distinct from being a chronic invalid confined to bed or armchair. A knowledge of the values of the blood gases in a patient suffering from chronic respiratory disease, prior to the episode which has resulted in the patient's present acute respiratory failure, will also help to act as a base line in assessing subsequent changes.

Initiating Artificial Ventilation

Having decided to ventilate a patient artificially, a ventilator is chosen and prepared for use. The following points are checked:

1. The ventilator must be clean with patient circuit sterilized. It must be connected to the mains and switched on if it is electrically operated.
2. Humidifier must be in circuit and filled and heated to required standards.
3. Oxygen must be connected and running to give required oxygen concentration in inspired mixture.
4. The rate, volume and/or pressure are set to desired levels.
5. The ventilator alarm (see Fig. 2.2) is set to signal at desired levels and incorporated into the circuit.

The ventilator tubing is then connected to the endotracheal tube or tracheostomy by appropriate connections, preferably using a swivel connection (see Fig. 2.3).

If the patient is 'fighting' the ventilator, i.e. his own respirations are asynchronous with the action of the ventilator or if he is anxious or in pain, intravenous analgesics such as

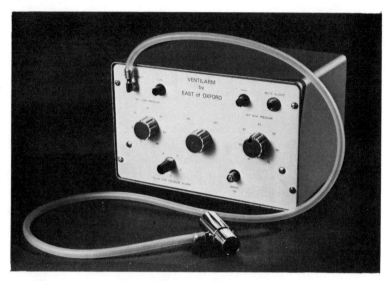

Fig. 2.2. Ventilator alarm with connection for inspiratory limb of circuit.

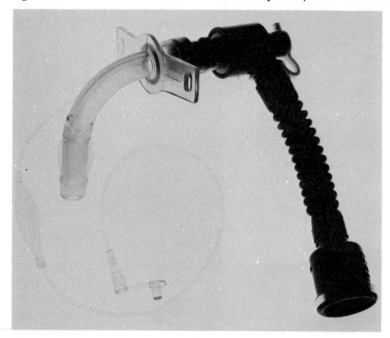

Fig. 2.3. Plastic tracheostomy tube with swivel connection to catheter mount.

phenoperidine (0·5—2 mg) or papaveretum (5—20 mg) may be given to settle him, and may be repeated as necessary. The side effect of respiratory depression which such analgesics possess is deliberately used in these cases, and this applies particularly to endotracheal tubes which are more uncomfortable for the patient than tracheostomy tubes.

Regulation of Artificial Ventilation

Close medical and nursing supervision is essential in order that artificial ventilation does not merely maintain life, but is continuously adjusted to the changing patterns of blood gas exchange and respiratory function which occur in the gravely ill.

In respiratory failure carbon dioxide elimination is impaired and physiological dead space is increased. Larger tidal volumes and minute volumes are consequently needed than would otherwise have been predicted from nomograms based only on physical characteristics. Tidal volumes of 600—850 and rates of 13—20 are used as initial calibrations for the ventilator.

Patterns of Ventilation. Although there is much written about different patterns and waveforms of ventilation, there are only a few points of practical importance.

Expiration should be longer than inspiration if cardiac output is to be maintained. A negative pressure should be avoided in order to prevent atelectasis. Tidal volumes, frequencies and percentages of oxygen in the inspiratory mixture are adjusted according to physical responses and blood gas estimations. A raised end expiratory pressure may sometimes be required (see later).

Blood gas estimations are performed to ensure that oxygenation and carbon dioxide elimination are satisfactory. These are needed more frequently in the early stages of artificial ventilation until a fairly stable state is reached. In those cases which require frequent arterial blood gas monitoring an indwelling arterial line may be used. This may be inserted into the radial, femoral or axillary arteries, the latter allowing greater mobility for the patient. Single samples are usually taken from the femoral artery using a heparinized glass syringe. PCO_2 levels should be maintained around normal physiological levels. In chronic lung disease the PCO_2 may be maintained at the usual elevated level. Values for PCO_2 should not be allowed to stay below 32 mm Hg for long periods since this may make weaning from the ventilator difficult. PCO_2 can be elevated by introducing an artificial mechanical dead space, or by adding carbon dioxide to the inspired gases. It is necessary to provide additional oxygen in the inspired mixture delivered by the ventilator, since patients in the Intensive Care Unit tend to have an increased alveolar-arterial oxygen tension difference. The percentage of oxygen in the inspired mixture is adjusted to give a PO_2 of between 75–100 mmHg. In conditions of anaemia, shock or lowered cardiac output it is necessary to provide more oxygen, and when in doubt to err on the side of a higher PO_2.

Various methods are available for improving the arterial oxygen tension, without necessarily increasing the percentage of oxygen in the inspired mixture. These include large tidal volumes, deep breaths every few minutes, and positive end expiratory pressure (PEEP) which provides continuous positive pressure within the lungs. All these methods help to prevent alveolar collapse. Positive end expiratory pressure improves arterial oxygenation without lowering the PCO_2. This is achieved by an attachment on the expiratory side of the patient circuit, which exerts back pressure on expiration. Severely ill patients with a low cardiac output may not be able to compensate for the cardiovascular changes brought about by continuous positive pressure.

Other investigations required will depend on the condition of the patient. They include:

Respiratory:	Chest X-ray.
	Sputum.
	Hb. & Hct.
	WBC.
Cardiovascular:	ECG.
	Cardiac output.
	Renal output.

Acid-Base Determinations: pH
(metabolic component of   Standard Bicarbonate
PCO_2 derangements)
Renal function tests.
Liver function tests.

Respiratory Failure

Nursing. All patients on ventilators should have constant nursing supervision.

½–1 hourly vital signs. P, BP, RR.

Hourly observations on the respirator volumes and pressures and oxygen concentrations in the inspired mixtures are maintained.

Daily water balance and weight observations are maintained to detect fluid retention.

The above observations together with 4-hourly temperature are recorded on a large chart, which is kept by the bedside. On a smaller 'flow chart' is kept results of investigations (see Acute renal failure chapter).

Ventilator alarms are checked frequently.

Secretions are aspirated as necessary, taking care to give 100% oxygen prior to suction when the PaO_2-PAO_2 difference is great. Aspiration should not exceed 15 seconds in duration.

Ventilator tubing is changed daily.

The humidifier is kept filled with sterile water.

Cuffs on endotracheal tubes and tracheostomy tubes are released every four hours for five minute intervals, and re-inflated until there is no leak.

Deep pulmonary inflations using an Ambu bag with oxygen are performed during periods of cuff release and during physiotherapy.

Sputum and tracheostomy stoma swabs are sent for culture and sensitivity daily.

Tracheostomy wound care 4–8 hourly as required.

Patients are repositioned 2-hourly.

Mouth and eye care in unconscious patients 4-hourly.

Where possible oral or tube feeds are provided.

Many patients need repeated reassurance and company whilst undergoing artificial ventilation. The nurse should explain the necessity for artificial ventilation to the patient and also that his inability to talk is only temporary. The conscious patient should have a pad and pencil to write with, and all procedures that disturb him should be explained. Similarly doctors who examine and treat the patient on a ventilator should also inform him of significant progress towards recovery.

Drugs. Various drugs are administered for the purpose of sedation and pain relief of patients receiving artificial ventilation. There are three indications for the use of potent analgesics or sedatives.

1. Pain.
2. Where respiratory efforts are being made which are asynchronous with those of the ventilator. An attempt should be made to eliminate insufficient artificial ventilation as the cause of the spontaneous respiratory efforts, before using drugs to suppress them. This can be done by trying the effects of large inflations with an Ambu bag or with the mechanical ventilator. See p. 85 (Insufficient ventilation).
3. When the patient is awake and anxious.

The drugs commonly used include:

Phenoperidine Morphine Papaveretum Pethidine	Analgesics
Diazepam Chlorpromazine Barbiturates	Tranquillizers and Sedatives
Tubocurarine Pancuronium	Muscle relaxants

These last agents are reserved for patients who are refractory to other drugs or who need absolute abolition of muscle activity. They should be combined with sedatives as the patient may be wide awake although paralysed.

Termination of Artificial Ventilation, and Weaning from the Ventilator

Obviously patients should not be artificially ventilated for longer periods than are necessary, since there are many hazards associated with the processes of artificial ventilation including those connected with the use of endotracheal tubes and tracheostomy tubes. Just as important but not always appreciated are the dangers of stopping artificial ventilation before the patient has recovered sufficiently to regain adequate pulmonary function and ventilatory reserve. The situation should not be allowed to occur in which a patient who has been artificially ventilated is then permitted to breathe spontaneously until over a period of some hours his condition deteriorates and he becomes exhausted and develops clinically obvious signs of respiratory failure. It is therefore necessary to try and decide in as accurate a manner as possible, the appropriate time to terminate artificial ventilation. Clinical response to artificial ventilation, antibiotics and other therapy will naturally have to be favourable before cessation of artificial ventilation is considered. It is seldom wise to cease artificial ventilation in the presence of other major system failure which could result in secondary pulmonary deterioration, for example the patient who has peritonitis or is in left ventricular failure. The age and previous health will sometimes influence the duration of artificial ventilation, thus young patients with chest trauma require shorter periods of mechanical ventilation than older patients.

Investigations.

See Table I
1. Disappearance of adverse radiological changes.
2. $PaO_2 - PAO_2$ differences.
3. $\dfrac{VD}{VT}$ Ratios.
4. VC (vital capacity).

Patients who have been ventilated for periods of less than two or three days and who were in good health prior to their acute respiratory failure will usually be able to be taken straight from the ventilator and allowed to breathe spontaneously. Those who have been ventilated for longer periods will need to be weaned from the mechanical ventilator by allowing increasing periods of time for spontaneous ventilation over a period of several days. Thus the period of spontaneous ventilation may start off at ten minutes per hour and increase to several hours at a time.

Respiratory depressant drugs should be avoided before the periods of spontaneous ventilation and additional humidified oxygen given via the tracheostomy or endotracheal tube during these periods, using a T-piece system. Throughout the weaning a close watch is kept on the pulse and respiratory rate, and blood gas values are checked towards the end of a period off the ventilator. After the patient is able to breathe unaided during the day he is taken off the ventilator at night.

It is never wise to try and hurry the weaning process. Undue exhaustion may lead to inefficient ventilation with alveolar collapse and infection, resulting in the patient having to return to continuous IPPV, and this apart from delaying medical recovery is also very bad for the morale of both the patient and nursing staff.

The tracheostomy tube should be retained for 24 hours after complete cessation of artificial ventilation. It is preferable to use a fenestrated tube at this stage, and this can be prepared by cutting an aperture in the plastic tube with a sterile scalpel blade. The proximal end of the tracheostomy tube may then be sealed off for 12 to 24 hours and if the patient is able to breathe adequately and cough up any secretions through his vocal cords, he may safely have his tube removed. A dry dressing is then placed over the stoma which heals rapidly.

Types of Artificial Mechanical Ventilator used in Intensive Care Units

A large and ever-increasing number of mechanical ventilators are available at present for use in Intensive Care Units. It is not necessary to understand the complexities of structure of such ventilators in order to use them effectively. The methods by which different ventilators bring about alternate inflation and deflation of the lungs have been classified in various ways. These classifications consider the component phases of inspiration and expiration and the two intervals between them in terms of pressure or volume achieved and the mechanism by which one phase is terminated and the next commenced (cycling). In clinical practice two types of ventilator are in common use in Intensive Care Units. These are pressure limited and volume limited ventilators.

Pressure limited ventilators. In these machines the pressure is pre-set so that if there are leaks in the circuit between the machine and the patient, inflation will continue till compensation occurs. Changes in compliance and airways resistance may however result in a decreased tidal volume being delivered by these machines since the pre-set pressure will be reached before the expected tidal volume has been provided. Examples of this type of ventilator include, Bird, Bennett, Radcliffe, Barnet and Blease. Certain of these ventilators can act as patient-triggered ventilators, inspiration being started by the patient's own efforts.

Volume limited ventilators. In these machines the volume is pre-set and the machine then delivers this volume, even though there may be changes in compliance or airways resistance in the lungs. When an excessive pressure is reached the gases leak out through a safety valve. Examples of this type of ventilator include the Cape, Cape—Bristol and the Engström.

Fig. 2.5 illustrates the Cape—Bristol ventilator which is in use in our Brighton Unit. This ventilator possesses amongst other advantages clearly understood dials, simply operated controls (of great value for nursing staff) and an autoclavable ventilating head which may be exchanged for a fresh ventilating circuit whilst being sterilized, so that the machine need never be out of action.

Ventilator Alarms and Respiratory Monitors. There are several alarms available which warn by lights and whistles that the pressure in the ventilatory circuit is either too high or too low. They will operate if there is obstruction or disconnection between the machine and the patient. An example of the type used in our unit is shown in Fig. 2.2.

Certain monitors alert the nurse should the frequency of spontaneous respirations exceed or fall below set limits and an example is shown in Fig. 2.4.

Sterilization of Ventilators. Ventilators that have become contaminated by bacterial pathogens can be sterilized by several techniques. These include:

Ethylene oxide,
Formalin vapour cabinets,

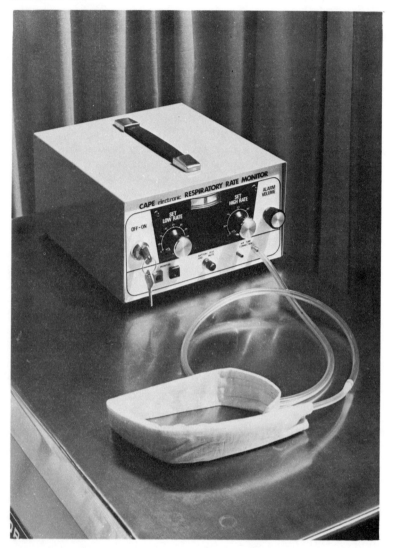

Fig. 2.4. Respiratory rate monitor with sensing sleeve which encircles thorax.

Autoclavable patient circuits as mentioned earlier, and Ultra-sonic nebulization with H_2O_2 or alcohol.

Bacterial filters are also used at inspiratory and outlet ports in an attempt to prevent contamination of the ventilator or

84

environment. Ventilator tubing can be disinfected by immersion in hot water or liquid disinfectant.

Complications of Artificial Mechanical Ventilation

The many complications of artificial mechanical ventilation should ensure that this treatment is not undertaken lightly. However, the gravity of the condition that is to be treated, i.e. respiratory failure, does not usually allow any prevarication in this matter. The potential complications of not supporting the respiratory processes either prophylactically or therapeutically during respiratory failure are themselves extensive and often lethal.

1. Those associated with the use of endotracheal tubes and tracheostomy tubes. See page 65.
2. Mechanical problems.

Familiarity with the chosen ventilator is of great importance, and simplicity in design of the operating controls (see Fig. 2.5) helps to reduce errors. Close monitoring of expiratory tidal volumes and inflation pressures and frequencies, gives early warning of changes in the lung. Disconnection or obstruction may occur and constant observation of tubing and connections is necessary, and ventilator alarms are an additional aid.

3. Disturbances of respiratory and cardiovascular function following mechanical ventilation.

(a) *Insufficient Ventilation.* Mechanical ventilators may be set to provide an inadequate volume of inspired gases for the patient's requirements. Atelectasis will tend to occur and the PCO_2 will rise and PO_2 fall. Should the percentage of oxygen in the inspired mixture be inadequate hypoxaemia will occur or be maintained. Either of these conditions can result in the patient attempting spontaneous ventilations ('fighting the ventilator'). Where 'fighting the ventilator' occurs the following should be checked:

(i) The cuff of the endotracheal tube or tracheostomy tube, to see that there are no leaks and so ensure the patient is receiving the expected inspiratory volume.
(ii) Tidal volume and frequency.

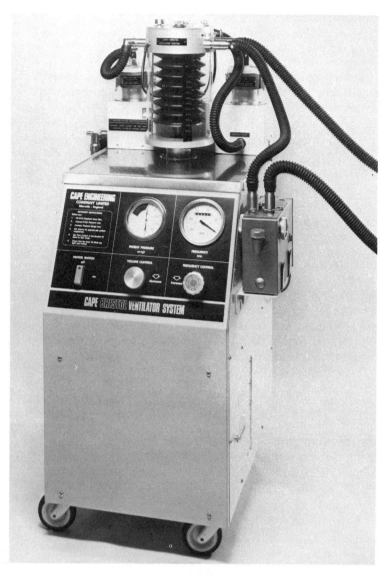

Fig. 2.5. CAPE-BRISTOL ventilator showing simplicity of dials and controls.

(iii) Percentage of oxygen in the inspired mixture. An immediate attempt should be made to give the patient adequate volumes and oxygenation by altering the ventilator settings or using an Ambu bag in the first instance. Only when these methods do not succeed is it necessary to give analgesics or sedatives to suppress the spontaneous respiratory efforts. Arterial blood, oxygen and carbon dioxide levels can be checked when there is any doubt as to the adequacy of artificial ventilation.

(b) *Over Ventilation*. Excessive tidal volumes result in a depression of PCO_2. This is useful in controlling attempts at spontaneous ventilations but if the PCO_2 is depressed for too long a period, below 32 mmHg, there may be some difficulty in getting a return of adequate spontaneous ventilations in weaning the patient from the ventilator. Pneumothorax may occur whilst a patient is receiving artificial ventilation, and is often associated with previous chest injury. Excessive inflation pressures are not a common cause of damage unless emphysematous bullae are present or there is gross airways obstruction, however a combination of large tidal volumes with positive end expiratory pressure may be dangerous. If the pneumothorax is large or a tension pneumothorax develops, a trocar and cannula should be inserted into the second intercostal space anteriorly on the affected side and a drain inserted and connected to an underwater seal, whilst artificial ventilation is continued.

(c) *Surgical Emphysema*. This is a distension of the subcutaneous tissues with air. The air may enter from the tracheostomy site or from a leak in the lower air passages. A delayed pneumothorax may present in this manner following the onset of artificial ventilation. A pneumothorax should be drained and any tracheostomy leak corrected. With continued mechanical ventilation, the distension may reach alarming proportions and incisions may be required when there is too great a pressure on the great veins or cardiac arrhythmias develop.

(d) *Pulmonary Oxygen Toxicity*. Histological changes have been observed in the lungs in patients who have received artificial ventilation together with high inspired concentrations of oxygen. However, several other causative factors may have been involved

87

in the development of such non-specific pathological changes as oedema, haemorrhage and hyaline membrane. From what evidence is available it seems that concentrations of oxygen of 0·6—1·0 atmospheres are likely to result in adverse pulmonary changes after 48 hours of continuous exposure and 70% concentration of oxygen in the inspired gases should not be exceeded unless it is impossible to maintain a suitably safe range of oxygen tensions in the arterial blood using intermittent positive pressure ventilation together with those techniques already discussed. In the event of severe hypoxaemia occurring in spite of the application of these measures, higher concentrations of oxygen should be given, since despite the danger of pulmonary oxygen toxicity the patient may succumb from systemic hypoxia long before pulmonary damage occurs. High oxygen concentrations should be reduced as fast as is compatible with maintaining reasonable arterial blood oxygen levels. It is believed that changes resulting from oxygen toxicity may be reversed if the high oxygen levels in the inspired mixture have not been maintained for too long a period.

(e) *Pulmonary Infection.* Although mechanical ventilators together with their tubing and humidifiers are a potential source of cross-infection, there is some doubt as to the extent to which they contribute to chest infections in the Intensive Care Unit. Certainly inadequate humidification and atelectasis both lead to pulmonary infection. Patients who are being artificially ventilated have endotracheal tubes or tracheostomy tubes, and even when organisms are cultured from the sputum, these are not always associated with clinical signs of infection. Gram negative organisms such as Proteus and Pseudomonas pyocyaneus are often found in the sputa of patients undergoing long term ventilation, especially after the use of wide spectrum antibiotics. It is hardly surprising that the debilitated patients who are being ventilated for a variety of reasons in the Intensive Care Unit frequently have chest infections and it may well be that effective expansion of alveoli by artificial ventilation is the best prophylactic against pulmonary infection.

(f) *Fluid Retention.* Prolonged artificial ventilation is associated with water retention and radiographic evidence of pulmonary oedema. This may respond to diuretic therapy and water restriction together with potassium replacement.

(g) *Cardiovascular Depression.* In the majority of patients receiving intermittent positive pressure ventilation, compensatory mechanisms rapidly adjust any tendency to a fall in cardiac output or lowering of the blood pressure. Positive end expiratory pressure sometimes results in an impaired cardiac output which may mask improvements in respiratory function.

In two groups of patients a rise in intra-thoracic and intra-pulmonary pressure as a result of mechanical ventilation may result in cardiovascular depression.

(i) Patients who are shocked with a lowered blood volume as after haemorrhage. A decrease in venous return due to a rise in intra-thoracic pressure may cause a fall in cardiac output in these patients. Similarly in those patients who already have a lowered cardiac output due to ischaemic changes following an infarct IPPV may result in further cardio-vascular depression.

(ii) Patients with asthma or obstructive airways disease have a prolonged expiration. In these patients, if there is any obstruction to expiration there will result an increase in the air trapped in the lungs with a resultant rise in intra-thoracic pressure and fall in venous return.

The hyperbaric oxygen chamber and the membrane oxygenator have both been used in an attempt to overcome problems associated with artificial mechanical ventilation.

As a result of an awareness of these various complications and the application of appropriate preventive measures, the survival rate following mechanical ventilation has improved considerably over recent years.

FURTHER READING
J. F. Nunn (1969). *Applied Respiratory Physiology.* Butterwoth & Co.
Bendixen, Egbert, Hedley-Whyte, Laver, Pontoppidan (1965). *Respiratory Care.* C. V. Mosby.
Mushin, Rendell-Baker, Thompson, Mapleson (1969). *Automatic Ventilation of the Lungs.* 2nd Edition. Blackwell.
Pontoppidan, Laver & Geffin (1970). Acute Respiratory Failure in the Surgical Patient in *Advances in Surgery*, 4, 163.
Sykes, McNicol, Campbell (1971). *Respiratory Failure.* Blackwell.

Chapter 3

Acute Renal Failure

PAUL SHARPSTONE

DIALYSIS

Indications

Principles

Haemodialysis

Peritoneal Dialysis

Choice of Haemodialysis or Peritoneal Dialysis

Technique of Peritoneal Dialysis

CLASSIFICATION

Acute renal failure is the sudden cessation or severe impairment of renal function. Its diagnosis in the early stages may be difficult since its most prominent features, a rise in blood urea concentration and a diminution of urine output, can both have other causes. The blood urea may be increased because of a rapid rate of urea production when there is excessive tissue breakdown in conditions such as severe sepsis, so that the kidneys, though functioning normally, are unable to excrete sufficient urea to prevent the blood level rising. The urine output falls in states of dehydration or other conditions in which renal blood flow is reduced, but unless this is severe, kidney function remains normal. Here the urine is highly concentrated, so that despite oliguria sufficient solute is excreted to keep the blood urea normal. When renal function is poor, however, the excretion of solute is impaired so that the blood urea rises even if tissue catabolism is not excessive. In acute renal failure there is usually, but not invariably, a reduction in urine volume as well.

Renal failure itself is divided into pre-renal, post-renal and intrinsic renal categories, and their distinction is vital since the former two can often be corrected, but if correction is delayed they may lead to intrinsic renal damage.

Physiological Oliguria

In dehydration of moderate degree a low urine output is physiological, and is distinguished from that of renal failure by the finding of a concentrated urine, i.e. specific gravity greater than

91

1022. Another simple test is to measure the urea concentration in both urine and blood. A ratio of urine to blood urea of greater than 10 indicates good renal function. Both of these tests are applicable only when there is oliguria (urine output less than 400 ml per 24 hours in an adult).

Pre-renal Failure

When hypovolaemia or hypotension is of more than moderate severity, the reduction of renal blood flow causes impairment of renal function so that waste products of metabolism accumulate in the body and produce the syndrome of uraemia. But the impairment may be functional and not associated with damage to the renal parenchyma, in which case it is described as pre-renal failure. The distinction between pre-renal and intrinsic renal failure is based upon the restoration of normal renal function in the former case as soon as the pre-renal factors have been corrected. The crude tests of urine concentrating ability give the same results in both conditions (Table I), and it follows that differentiation between them is usually made retrospectively. The difficulty of prospective diagnosis is of no great importance since it is essential to correct pre-renal factors rapidly even if there is intrinsic renal failure.

TABLE I Urinary Concentrating Ability and the Response
to Treatment in Oliguric States

Condition	Effect of correction of precipitating factor	Urine specific gravity	Urine/plasma urea ratio	Effect of Mannitol
Physiological oliguria	Reversed	> 1022	> 10	Reversed
Pre-renal failure				
Intrinsic renal failure	Not reversed	< 1022	< 10	Not reversed

Intrinsic Renal Failure

In these conditions there is organic renal damage and renal failure persists even if the precipitating factors are corrected. However, in some patients with incipient acute tubular necrosis mannitol given at an early stage will reverse the oliguria.

Post-renal Failure

This occurs when there is severe or complete obstruction of the urinary tract anywhere between the renal calyces and the external urethral meatus. Post renal obstruction may sometimes cause acute renal failure (e.g. the impaction of a calculus in the ureter of a solitary kidney), but much more commonly it produces slowly progressive renal failure. However, chronic obstructive uropathy, like other varieties of chronic renal failure, may present as advanced uraemia with little or no past history of renal symptoms, thus mimicking acute renal failure. Therefore the possibility of obstruction must be considered in every patient.

CAUSES OF ACUTE RENAL FAILURE

Table II lists the commoner causes of acute renal failure. The intrinsic renal conditions require further discussion.

Acute Tubular Necrosis

This syndrome is caused by ischaemic or toxic injury to the kidney and is characterized by the abrupt cessation of renal function and spontaneous recovery, usually within three weeks, if the patient survives that long. The histological changes in the kidney include necrosis of proximal tubular epithelium, blood casts in the tubules and interstitial oedema, but the changes are often not very pronounced and the reason for the oliguria persisting long after the original insult has ceased is unknown.

Acute tubular necrosis is probably the most important condition requiring dialysis since efficient control of uraemia until the renal lesion recovers will result in the survival of a patient who has essentially normal renal function.

TABLE II Causes of Acute Renal Failure

Pre-renal

Hypovolaemia or hypotension	Haemorrhage Plasma loss (e.g. burns) Dehydration Septicaemic shock Cardiogenic shock Sedative drug overdose

Intrinsic Renal Failure

Acute Tubular Necrosis

Ischaemic	Any pre-renal cause if severe and prolonged

Nephrotoxic	Haemoglobinaemia (e.g. incompatible
	  blood transfusions)
	Myoglobinaemia (e.g. crush injury)
	Bacterial toxin (e.g. Cl. welchii
	  septicaemia)
	Paracetamol overdose
	Carbon tetrachloride
	Ethylene glycol
	Heavy metals

Bilateral Cortical Necrosis

Glomerulonephritis

Post-streptococcal acute glomerulonephritis
Rapidly progressive glomerulonephritis
Multi-system disease (polyarteritis nodosa,
        SLE, Goodpasture's
        syndrome, etc.)

Miscellaneous

Malignant hypertensive nephrosclerosis
Weil's disease
Allergic interstitial nephritis (e.g. phen-
        indione)
Thrombotic thrombocytopenic purpura
Haemolytic-uraemic syndrome
Fulminating acute pyelonephritis
Papillary necrosis
Osmotic diuretic nephropathy
Pre-eclampsia
Sulphonamide crystalluria
Hypercalcaemia
Urate nephropathy
Renal vein or artery occlusion

TABLE II (*continued*)

Post-renal

Calculus obstruction of solitary kidney
Pelvic-ureteric obstruction
Retroperitoneal fibrosis'
Malignant pelvic or retroperitoneal tumour
Prostatic hypertrophy
Urethral stricture

Any of the causes of pre-renal failure, particularly if severe or prolonged, may result in ischaemia of the kidneys severe enough to lead to acute tubular necrosis. In addition, a variety of nephrotoxins may be responsible. These include haemoglobin (as in incompatible blood transfusions or black water fever), myoglobin (crush injury, burns), bacterial toxins (Clostridium welchii septicaemia, septic abortions), and various exogenous toxins, some of which are listed in Table II. Susceptibility to acute tubular necrosis is increased in pregnancy, cirrhosis of the liver with ascites, advanced cardiac failure, the nephrotic syndrome, severe liver failure, and obstructive jaundice. For example, quite modest blood loss from an antepartum haemorrhage is much more likely to cause renal failure than a haemorrhage of similar magnitude in a non-pregnant patient.

Bilateral Cortical Necrosis

A minority of patients with acute renal failure developing in the same circumstances as acute tubular necrosis sustain a more severe degree of renal damage known as bilateral cortical necrosis. This is irreversible and, though a patchy lesion, is often widespread, so that useful renal function may not be regained. Sometimes it can be diagnosed by the finding of calcification in the renal cortices on X-ray examination, but more often it is suspected only when a patient with acute renal failure fails to recover after four weeks. Its most common cause is a haemorrhagic accident of late pregnancy in a patient with pre-eclampsia.

Glomerulonephritis

The acute renal failure of post-streptococcal acute glomerulonephritis is usually transient, and dialysis is only exceptionally

95

required for its control. Renal failure caused by other types of glomerulonephritis is usually chronic, but some have a rapidly progressive course leading to end-stage renal failure within a few weeks of onset. The most common variety of rapidly progressive glomerulonephritis affects mainly middle-aged and elderly patients and is associated with large epithelial crescents in the glomeruli leading to obliteration of the glomerular tufts. A similar course is sometimes produced by the renal lesions of certain multi-system diseases.

When oliguria due to glomerulonephritis lasts for more than a few days recovery of useful renal function is exceptional.

Miscellaneous

The vascular, allergic, infective, toxic and metabolic conditions listed in Table II cause acute renal failure by a variety of pathological mechanisms.

Exacerbation of Chronic Renal Failure

In a patient presenting with uraemia, an exacerbation of pre-existing chronic renal disease must always be considered in the differential diagnosis. Common precipitating factors are an intercurrent illness, such as an infection or surgical operation, resulting in a reduction of fluid intake, which in turn aggravates the uraemia. A vicious circle is easily started, with uraemic anorexia and vomiting leading to further dehydration and impairment of already precarious renal function. The importance of making the correct diagnosis here is that, though it may be impossible to do anything for the underlying renal disease, correction of the extra-renal disturbance will often restore renal function to its previous level, and perhaps allow the patient several more years of reasonable existence.

DIAGNOSTIC APPROACH

History

The first step is to establish whether there is any previous history of symptoms of renal tract disease, such as 'cystitis', haematuria, loin pain, difficulty in micturition, or of symptoms suggestive of renal failure, such as nocturia and thirst. The less specific symptoms of anorexia, nausea and vomiting are also suggestive. A record of proteinuria or hypertension in the past is, of course, indicative of chronic renal disease. The family history is important, since some varieties of renal disease are inherited. For example, a history of relatives dying of renal failure in middle life would be very suggestive of polycystic disease.

Next, it is necessary to enquire carefully into the circumstances of the onset of the present illness. Acute tubular necrosis usually has a clear-cut onset at the time of some catastrophe such as a haemorrhage, septicaemia or a severe hypotensive episode during or after a surgical operation. But a nephrotoxic cause may not be so obvious. For example, a patient may not recognize the significance of his having inhaled carbon tetrachloride some days previously. A history of analgesic abuse is often not revealed spontaneously.

The records of a patient who develops renal failure while in hospital must be examined in detail; fluid input and output charts may demonstrate a deficit, or a hypotensive episode may be identified, pointing to a pre-renal cause of uraemia.

An asymptomatic onset of renal failure suggests glomerulonephritis as the cause. In post-renal uraemia a history of difficulty of micturition, intermittent polyuria and oliguria, or pain in the back or loins may be obtained. If there is complete anuria, obstruction of the renal tract is very likely.

Examination

The state of the patient's circulation and hydration should be assessed with particular attention to skin turgor, jugular venous pressure, the lung bases, and oedema. Dryness of the tongue may be misleading, since mouth breathing may be the cause, especially when there is hyperventilation. The signs of advanced uraemia, such as drowsiness, acidotic respiration, bruising and a pericardial friction rub should be looked for. Chronic renal failure is suggested by skin pigmentation, wasting, severe anaemia without other cause, and dehydration. In prostatic or urethral obstruction, the bladder will be distended, while renal

swellings may be palpable in obstruction higher up. In polycystic disease, enlargement of the kidneys will be found. Rectal
examination should never be omitted since prostatic enlargement and pelvic tumours are important causes of obstructive
uraemia. The bladder should be catheterized to exclude lower
urinary tract obstruction, but unless this is present the catheter
should be removed at once since it is especially likely to cause
sepsis when there is a poor urine flow. When malignant hypertension is the cause of renal failure, a severe retinopathy will be
found, though it is often difficult to decide whether malignant
hypertension is the result or the cause of renal disease. In
glomerulonephritis associated with multi-system disease clues
may be obtained from extra-renal features, such as the facial
rash of systemic lupus erythematosus, the purpura of Henoch—
Schonlein disease, or neuropathy in polyarteritis nodosa.

Finally, when acute tubular necrosis occurs without an
apparently sufficient cause undiagnosed complications of the
primary illness should be suspected: for example, the development of biliary peritonitis after an apparently uncomplicated
cholecystectomy, a gangrenous uterus after abortion, or the
ligation of ureters at hysterectomy.

Investigations

The initial investigations to be carried out on all patients are
listed in Table III. A particularly valuable test to distinguish
between acute tubular necrosis and pre-renal failure is the finding of a urine sodium concentration greater than 40 mEq/1 in
the former. Red blood cells and granular casts in large quantities
in the urine usually indicate glomerulonephritis but are sometimes found in acute tubular necrosis. They do not occur, however, in obstructive renal failure.

A plain X-ray of the abdomen is a most important investigation. It will reveal radio-opaque calculi and, in addition, in films
of good quality, will often show the renal outlines. If necessary
tomography of the renal areas should be carried out as well.
Small kidneys are diagnostic of long-standing renal disease,
though they are not invariably found.

Other investigations which are needed in particular patients
only include the following:

TABLE III Investigations

All Patients

Blood	Hb, WBC, Platelets, Film
	Urea, sodium, potassium, bicarbonate
	Creatinine
	Calcium, phosphate
	Proteins
	Culture
Urine	Specific gravity or osmolality
	Protein concentration
	Microscopy for RBC's, WBC's and casts
	Culture
	Urea
	Sodium
X-rays	Chest
	Abdomen
ECG	

Selected Patients

High dose IVP
Cystoscopy and retrograde pyelography
Renal biopsy
Renal arteriogram
Renal venogram

Intravenous Pyelogram. The intravenous pyelogram can produce valuable information in advanced renal failure if a sufficiently high dose of the contrast medium is used, and tomography carried out if necessary. A dose of 2 ml per kilogram body weight of Hypaque 45% is given intravenously by syringe — drip infusion is unnecessary — and films taken immediately, at five minutes, ten minutes, thirty minutes, one hour, and at intervals up to twenty-four hours as necessary. In most cases sufficient detail can be seen to define the shape and size of the kidneys and exclude or confirm the presence of extra-renal obstruction.

Retrograde Pyelography. Obstruction of the renal tract must be considered in every case of acute renal failure unless another cause is obvious. The high dose intravenous pyelogram has lessened the need for retrograde pyelography but not eliminated it, and if obstruction has not been positively excluded, cysto-scopy and retrograde pyelography should be carried out.

Renal Biopsy. Renal biopsy is necessary when glomerulone-phritis or other intrinsic causes of acute renal failure are sus-pected, unless the diagnosis is evident from the extra-renal manifestations of the disease. It is not required in acute tubular necrosis unless oliguria has persisted for four weeks or longer. Uraemia should be controlled by dialysis before biopsy is under-taken, and other prerequisites are a normal prothrombin time and platelet count, the absence of severe hypertension, and the radiological demonstration of two kidneys of normal or nearly normal size.

Many other investigations may be required in individual patients: for example, renal arteriography, renal venography, plasma and urine spectroscopy for haemoglobin and myoglobin, antinuclear factor and LE cells tests.

MANAGEMENT

Phrophylaxis and Treatment of the Renal Lesion

Correction of Pre-renal Factors. The most important measure by far for the prevention of acute tubular necrosis is to correct pre-renal factors as rapidly and completely as possible. Sometimes hypotension cannot be reversed, as in cardiogenic shock, but in most cases there is reduction in the volume of fluid in the intra-vascular bed. This may be the result of loss of fluid outside the body as in diarrhoea and vomiting or the plasma loss in burns, or sequestration of fluid within the body outside the vascular compartment. Examples of the latter are: in the gut in ileus, in the peritoneal cavity in peritonitis, or in the soft tissues around the site of a major injury. In other cases the absolute volume of intravascular fluid is normal, but there is a deficiency relative to an expanded capacity of the vascular bed in conditions such as gram — negative septicaemia and barbiturate poisoning. In every case the mainstay of treatment is the replacement of fluid in sufficient quantity.

The type of fluid used will depend on what is lost. For

100

example, normal saline is required for loss of gastro-intestinal secretion, blood for haemorrhage, and plasma for burns. Large volumes are often required and a common mistake is to interpret the oliguria of dehydration as indicating renal failure and to restrict the fluid input, with consequent exacerbation of renal failure. It may be difficult to distinguish pre-renal and intrinsic renal failure prospectively, but even in the latter pre-renal factors must be corrected as rapidly as possible.

The volume of fluid to be given must be assessed from clinical criteria such as the previous fluid input and output charts, the level of the blood pressure, and the skin turgor. Circulatory overload must be avoided by careful observation of the jugular venous pressure and auscultation for crepitations at the lung bases. Peripheral oedema indicates an excess of extra-cellular fluid but not necessarily of intravascular fluid; in hypoproteinaemic states such as the nephrotic syndrome and cirrhosis of the liver there is often hypovolaemia despite oedema. These states should be corrected with a plasma expander which remains within the vascular compartment, such as Dextran 70 or plasma.

If large volumes of fluid are to be infused rapidly a useful safeguard is to monitor the central venous pressure with a simple manometer connected to a catheter in the superior vena cava. (see Chapter 7). The absolute level of central venous pressure is of less importance than the change induced by treatment. Infusion can be continued with reasonable safety until the level begins to rise. The central venous pressure, however, should not be relied upon to the exclusion of other observations, since left ventricular failure can occur without a rise in the right heart pressure.

Mannitol. Mannitol has been shown to prevent the development of acute tubular necrosis in some patients, if given early enough after the provoking incident. As soon as pre-renal failure has been treated, 200 ml of a 10% solution of mannitol should be given intravenously in ten minutes. If the urine flow rate increases to over 40 ml per hour, further doses should be given as necessary to maintain an output of about 100 ml per hour. Frusemide is probably equally effective and is a simpler-to-use alternative to mannitol. It should be given in doses of 40 mg intravenously, though much higher doses have been used with

101

success. Mannitol may also be used prophylactically in situations in which there is a high risk of renal failure developing —
for example, in operations on patients with deep obstructive
jaundice and in surgery of the aorta. An infusion of 5% mannitol
should be started pre-operatively.

Established Renal Failure. Once acute tubular necrosis is
established no treatment is available for the renal lesion;
spontaneous recovery of renal function within three or four
weeks may be expected, if the patient survives until then.

If acute renal failure due to glomerulonephritis lasts more
than a few days recovery of useful renal function is unlikely.
Earlier enthusiasm for immunosuppressive and anticoagulant
drugs in oliguric glomerulonephritis is waning but their use is
still under trial and these patients should have the benefit of an
expert nephrological opinion as early as possible in the course
of their disease. In any case, dialysis should be continued for at
least six weeks, and if possible, the patient transferred to a
maintenance haemodialysis programme. Specific therapy,
however, is available for some of the other causes of acute renal
parenchymal disease: for example, antihypertensives in hypertensive nephrosclerosis, penicillin in Weil's disease, prednisone in
hypercalcaemia, antibiotics in acute pyelonephritis, and allo-
purinol in urate nephropathy. Obstruction of the urinary tract
is usually amenable to surgery, but dialysis may be required to
prepare the patient for operation.

General Measures

Now that effective means are available to control uraemia the
outcome for patients with acute tubular necrosis is largely
determined by the severity of the underlying disease. The
mortality ranges from about 15 per cent when it is due to
incompatible blood transfusion or a nephrotoxin to more than
70 per cent in burns and major trauma. This emphasizes the
need for as intensive treatment of associated disorders as of the
renal failure. It is no use dialyzing a patient with acute renal
failure due to a septic abortion if a gangrenous uterus remains
in situ. The full resources of an intensive care unit are usually
required and it is essential to ensure close collaboration between

the various specialists involved in the care of the patient. As with other very sick patients, the quality of nursing care and physiotherapy is of crucial importance, particularly for the prevention of decubitus ulcers, oral sepsis and chest complications.

Uraemic patients are particularly susceptible to infection and sepsis is a common cause of death. Prophylactic antibiotics are undesirable but infection should be sought and treated early and vigorously. Antibiotics eliminated by the kidney, even toxic ones, need not be avoided provided the dose is appropriately reduced (Table IV). Tetracycline and chloramphenicol, however, should never be used when renal function is impaired, since the former can aggravate uraemia, and toxic metabolites of the latter can accumulate.

Care must be taken not to overlook the patient's emotional needs, and time must be taken to give explanation and

TABLE IV Dosage of Antibacterial Agents in Oliguric Renal Failure

Degree of dose reduction	Drug	Intervals at which Standard dose should be given
Major (check serum level if used for more than a week)	Streptomycin	3–4 days
	Gentamicin	3–4 days
	Kanamycin	3–4 days
	Colistin	2–3 days
	Vancomycin	2 weeks
Minor	Benzylpenicillin	8 hours
	Ampicillin	12 hours
	Cloxacillin	8 hours
	Carbenicillin	8 hours
	Cephaloridine	24 hours
	Cephalexin	24 hours
	Lincomycin	12 hours
None	Sodium fusidate	As in normal renal function
	Doxycycline	
	Nalidixic acid	
Avoid in renal failure	Tetracycline	—
	Chloramphenicol	
	Nitrofurantoin	

reassurance about the strange and frightening procedures to which he is being subjected.

Laboratory measurements which must be made each day include: blood urea, sodium, potassium, bicarbonate and haemoglobin. The control of treatment is made very much easier if these results, together with other relevant investigations, and the patient's weight, urine output and fluid intake are entered each day on a simple flow sheet (Fig. 3.1). The temptation to leave a catheter in place in the bladder to measure the urine output accurately should be resisted unless there is lower urinary tract obstruction. The onset of diuresis will soon become evident without its aid.

Treatment of Uraemia

Fluid and Electrolyte Intake. The aim is to maintain the volume and composition of the body fluid as close to normal as possible. During oliguria the excretion of water, sodium, potassium and nitrogenous products is negligible, so their intake must be curtailed.

The average adult loses about 1000 ml of water each day by routes other than the kidney, i.e. lungs, skin and gastro-intestinal tract. But some 600 ml of water are produced by tissue catabolism, so the basic daily water requirement for the anuric adult patient is 400 ml. To this must be added a volume of fluid equal to that of urine passed, and of any loss from the gastro-intestinal tract in vomiting or diarrhoea. An additional allowance should be given if there is fever or hyperventilation. A careful fluid input and output chart should be kept, but the most reliable guide to overall fluid balance is the patient's weight, which should be measured each day if possible. Some loss of tissue mass is inevitable during the course of acute renal failure, so the patient's weight should fall by about 0·3 kg per day, otherwise he is probably being overloaded with fluid.

No electrolyte should be given while the urine output remains low, except to compensate for overt loss. Though many patients have a low serum sodium concentration, this is usually due to dilution of a normal body sodium content by an excess of water, and no attempt should be made to correct it by giving sodium.

During the recovery phase of acute tubular necrosis the urine

ACUTE RENAL FAILURE

DATE				
URINE OUTPUT				
FLUID IN				
WEIGHT				
BLOOD UREA				
SODIUM				
POTASSIUM				
BICARBONATE				
Hb				
P.C.V.				
WBC				
PROTEIN				
HD				
P D VOL				
P D BALANCE				

Fig. 3.1. Part of acute renal failure flow-sheet.

output increases rapidly and may reach several litres per day. The renal function remains poor and, in particular, the kidney is unable to conserve water and electrolytes. At this stage correspondingly large amounts of fluid, sodium and potassium must be given to avoid depletion.

Nutrition. An adequate calorie intake is needed to avoid ketosis and excessive tissue breakdown, which would aggravate the

105

acidosis and uraemia. Since fluid, electrolytes and protein must be restricted, a concentrated solution of dextrose is usually used. The most palatable form of this is Hycal (Beechams), a flavoured liquid dextrose concentrate, four bottles of which provide 1700 calories with only 400 ml of water. Many patients are unable to tolerate even Hycal in these quantities and a useful supplement is Caloreen (Scientific Hospital Supplies), a soluble glucose polymer, which is less sweet. Vitamin supplements should be given. Many patients are unable to take an oral diet because of anorexia, vomiting, ileus, peritonitis or gastro-intestinal fistula. Their nutrition must be maintained by the intravenous route, using 20% dextrose solution. Higher concentrations lead to thrombophlebitis and if the daily input is limited to 500 ml only 400 calories will be provided by this means. This is barely adequate, but fortunately the availability of dialysis makes stringent dietary restriction of this sort rarely necessary for very long.

Hyperkalaemia. The most dangerous complication of acute renal failure is potassium intoxication. When the serum potassium is greater than 7·0 mEq/1, cardiac arrest may occur at any time. The characteristic electrocardiographic changes (Fig. 3.2), provide a more reliable warning than the serum level. Hyperkalaemia is controlled by the oral or rectal administration of 30 gm of calcium resonium, a resin which exchanges calcium for potassium in the gut. Its effect is not immediate and life-threatening potassium intoxication must be corrected more quickly by the intravenous infusion of 100 mEq of sodium bicarbonate, or with insulin 20 units subcutaneously along with glucose 60 gm intravenously.

Hypercatabolic State. The rate of rise of blood urea in patients without renal function is determined by the rate of endogenous protein breakdown and the amount of protein ingested. It ranges from 20 mg/100 ml per day in patients who are well apart from their renal failure and are taking an optimum diet, to 100 mg/100 ml per day in patients whose renal failure is associated with major trauma, burns or sepsis (Fig. 3.3). A daily rise of more than 60 mg/100 ml indicates a hypercatabolic state, and in this condition hyperkalaemia and acidosis may develop with

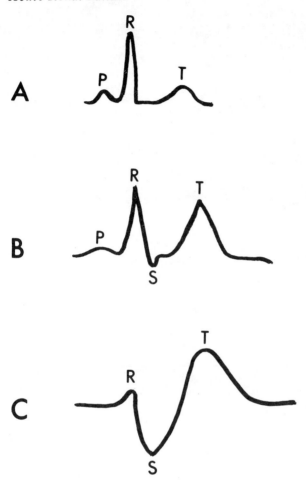

Fig. 3.2. The ECG in hyperkalaemia. A, normal trace. B, moderately severe hyperkalaemia, showing low amplitude P wave, prolonged P—R interval, increased width of QRS complex and a tall pointed T wave. C, severe hyperkalaemia, showing loss of P wave, reduction of R wave, deep S wave, and ST segment continuous with ascending limb of T wave.

alarming rapidity. It follows therefore that some patients with non-hypercatabolic renal failure may be maintained in reasonable health for up to two weeks by dietary manipulation alone, whereas patients with hypercatabolic states can die from uraemia within a few days of onset unless dialysis is used.

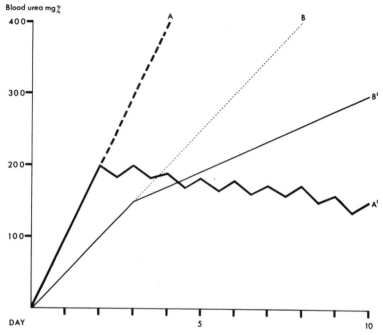

Fig. 3.3. Rate of rise of blood urea in hypercatabolic and non-hypercatabolic renal failure, and the effect of treatment.
A, hypercatabolic state. A[1] hypercatabolic state treated with peritoneal dialysis. B, non-hypercatabolic state. B[1], non-hypercatabolic state treated with dietary protein restriction.

DIALYSIS

Indications

Death from uraemia is imminent when the blood urea is greater than 400 mg per 100 ml, the serum potassium greater than 7·0 mEq/1 or bicarbonate less than 10 mEq/1, but even when the biochemical disturbance is less extreme, the patient is still at risk from sepsis, haemorrhage, fluid overload, failure of wound healing and malnutrition. Therefore, dialysis should be looked upon as a means of preventing rather than treating uraemia, and should be used early and vigorously. As a general guide, dialysis

108

should be started when the blood urea is about 200 mg per
100 ml, but more reliance should be placed on clinical rather
than biochemical criteria. In a well, non-hypercatabolic patient
in whom early recovery is expected, the blood urea may be
allowed to rise a little higher, whereas dialysis should be started
earlier in a hypercatabolic patient, or if there is circulatory
overload. The aim should be to keep the blood urea less than
200 mg per 100 ml at all times, and in a hypercatabolic patient
this may necessitate haemodialysis every day.

Once dialysis has been started fluid, salt and protein restriction should be relaxed, so that an almost normal diet or full
parenteral nutrition (see Chapter 9) can be given.

Principles of Dialysis

The patient's blood is passed across one surface of a semi-
permeable membrane, whose other surface is bathed in an
aqueous fluid, the dialysate. This is a solution of salts in
concentrations corresponding to those of normal plasma, with
the exception of potassium which is absent or low. The dialysate also contains glucose to render it hypertonic to plasma.
Crystalloid solutes diffuse freely across the membrane in the
direction of their concentration gradients. Thus urea and other
nitrogenous waste products and potassium, which are present
in the plasma but not in the dialysate, are washed out (Fig. 3.4).
At the same time the concentrations of plasma electrolytes such
as sodium and calcium, which are often low in uraemia, are
corrected by diffusion in from the dialysate. Water is removed
from the plasma by hydrostatic or by osmotic pressure, and the
amount removed may be controlled by adjusting the pressure
gradient across the membrane or the osmotic concentration of
the dialysate. The size of the membrane pores is such that blood
cells and protein molecules are not lost from the blood, and
bacteria cannot enter from the dialysate (though bacterial toxins
can).

Haemodialysis

Access to the circulation is obtained by the insertion of cannulae
in a peripheral artery (usually the radial) and vein. Between

109

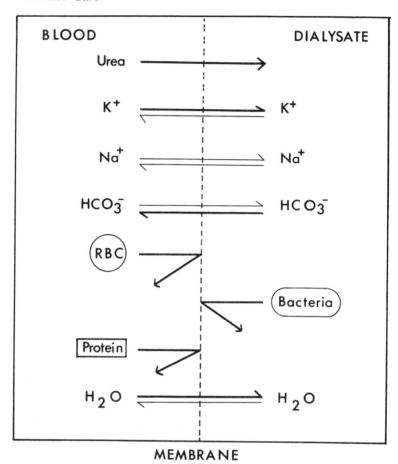

Fig. 3.4. The principles of dialysis.

dialyses the cannulae are kept opened by connecting them to each other as an external arterio-venous shunt. The dialysis membrane is made of cellophane or a similar substance and is constructed either as a coil of flat tubing through which the blood is pumped, or as a sandwich of two sheets in apposition, between which the blood flows under arterial pressure. The rest of the artificial kidney is simply an arrangement to store or produce the dialysis fluid and pump it at body temperature over the outer surface of the membrane. Heparin is used to prevent clotting in the extracorporeal circuit.

110

Peritoneal Dialysis

Here the dialysis membrane is the peritoneal membrane, the blood supply is the underlying capillary network and the dialysate reservoir is the peritoneal cavity (Fig. 3.5). The dialysate is introduced and drained by a catheter inserted through the anterior abdominal wall.

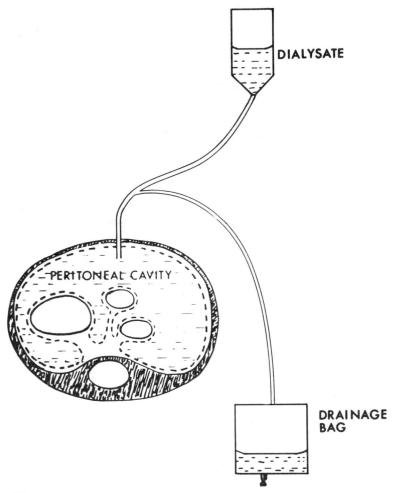

Fig. 3.5. Diagram of peritoneal dialysis.

Choice of Haemodialysis or Peritoneal Dialysis

Table V gives the advantages and drawbacks of each technique, and these should be considered when the choice is made for each patient. Well-closed recent abdominal wounds are not a contra-indication to peritoneal dialysis, nor is peritonitis or pancreatitis,

TABLE V Comparison of Haemodialysis and Peritoneal Dialysis

	Haemodialysis	Peritoneal dialysis
Specialized equipment and technical expertize needed	Much	Little
Time to set up	c.2 hours	c.15 mins
Efficiency of dialysis	High	Low
Complications	'Disequilibrium syndrome' Acute blood loss from rupture of extra-corporeal circuit Air embolus Haemorrhagic state from heparin	Trauma to abdominal viscera Peritonitis Respiratory embarrassment Discomfort to patient Loss of plasma protein
Contraindications	When systemic heparin is dangerous	Obliteration of peritoneal cavity by previous major surgery Intra-peritoneal drains Ventilatory insufficiency

which themselves may be benefited by peritoneal lavage. Though peritoneal dialysis can control uraemia in even severly hyper-catabolic states, it is less efficient than haemodialysis and may need to be continuous for a longer period. In this condition, intermittent haemodialysis is usually preferable. The high efficiency of haemodialysis can be a drawback since the too rapid removal of urea from a patient with advanced uraemia may produce a disequilibrium syndrome due to osmotic shifts between the brain and the extracellular fluid. When there is a relative or absolute contraindication to peritoneal dialysis, the patient should be transferred at an early stage to a unit with facilities for haemodialysis, rather than waiting for complications to develop or uraemia to get out of control.

However, in the majority of patients, both techniques are equally suitable. Since peritoneal dialysis is more readily available, it is more widely used. But though relatively simple it is dangerous unless carried out correctly and should not be undertaken without prior experience under supervision.

Technique of Peritoneal Dialysis

Table VI lists the equipment required and its suppliers.

TABLE VI Equipment for Peritoneal Dialysis

Item	Manufacturer and UK distributor	Specification	Remarks
Catheter	Allen and Hanburys Ltd. London E.2	Dialaflex Mk. 2	Semi-rigid
	Baxter Laboratories Ltd. Thetford, Norfolk	Diacath	With protective sleeve and adhesive disc
	Mcgaw Laboratories Inc. Chas. F. Thackray Park St., Leeds	Trocath Adult Size Trocath Paediatric Size	Semi-rigid
	B. Braun Melsugen Armour Pharmaceutical Co. Ltd. Eastbourne, Sussex	2·5 x 3·5 x 280 mm (adult) 1·5 x 2·7 x 200 mm (paediatric)	Flexible
Administration Set	Allen and Hanburys Ltd. Baxter Laboratories Ltd.	Dialaflex giving set Dianeal administration set	
Drainage bag	Aldington Laboratories Ltd. Mersham, Ashford, Kent Baxter Laboratories Ltd.	Aldon 3-litre drainage bag with outlet 3-litre drainage bag	
Dialysate	Allen and Hanburys Ltd.	Dialaflex 61 (dextrose 1·36%) Dialaflex 62 (dextrose 6·36%) Dialaflex 63 (dextrose 1·36% Na 130 mEq/1)	Collapsible plastic container

Boots Pure Drug Co. Ltd. Nottingham	Difusor 1·36% Difusor 6·36%	Semi-rigid plastic container
Baxter Laboratories Ltd.	Dianeal A 5204 (dextrose 1·5%) Dianeal A 5254 (dextrose 1·5% Na 130 mEq/1) Dianeal A 5961 (dextrose 1·5% Na 130 mEq/1 K 2·5 mEq/1)	Glass bottles

Insertion of Catheter. Before insertion of the peritoneal catheter, the bladder must be emptied. The preferred site is the relatively avascular mid-line, one third of the way from the umbilicus to the pubis, but any site on the anterior abdominal wall may be used, provided that the vicinity of operation scars and enlarged viscera is avoided. Local anaesthesia must be generous and about 10 ml of 1% Lignocaine should be injected intradermally, sub-cutaneously and deeply down to the peritoneum. A stab incision is made with a number 15 scalpel blade. The patient is asked to raise his head from the bed in order to tense his abdominal muscles and the catheter is inserted by means of its stylet (Fig. 3.6).

Though the pressure on the stylet must be controlled to avoid perforating deep structures it needs to be quite firm to penetrate the abdominal wall. The most common mistake is to leave the tip of the catheter too superficial, so that dialysate is infused into extra-peritoneal tissues. Once through the abdominal wall the catheter is angled inferiorly and pushed over the stylet until its tip is in the pelvis. The stylet is withdrawn and the dialysate giving-set connected. It is important to infuse some dialysate immediately to prevent blockage of the catheter holes by blood clot. In unconscious patients, young children and others unable to tense the abdominal muscles, the peritoneal cavity is disten-ded before insertion of the catheter by one litre of dialysate infused via a lumbar puncture needle. A pursestring suture is not required around the catheter. The site is covered with a gauze dressing and the free end of the catheter is taped securely

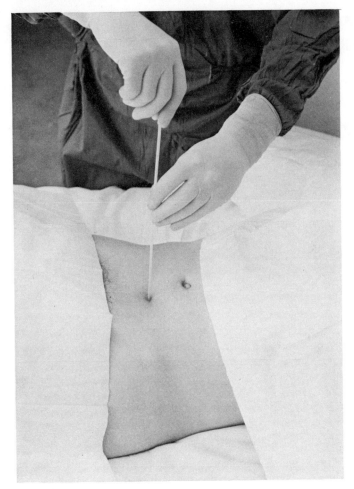

Fig. 3.6. Insertion of peritoneal dialysis catheter.

to the skin (Fig. 3.7). Even the semi-rigid catheters can be secured this way and flanges and other devices to maintain the catheter perpendicular to the abdominal wall are unnecessary.

Infusion of Dialysate. The dialysate is warmed prior to use in a basin of hot water, or, preferably, in a warming cabinet. Heparin 1000 units per litre is added to each of the first three exchanges to prevent blockage of the catheter by fibrin, but is

115

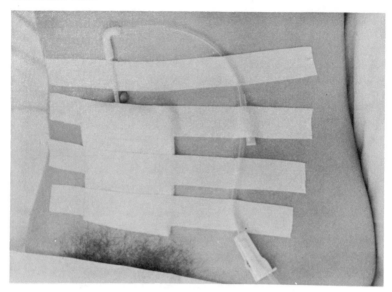

Fig. 3.7. Securing of peritoneal dialysis catheter.

not needed subsequently unless the dialysate remains blood-stained. Antibiotics are not used routinely in the dialysate. The commercially available dialysate contains no potassium and when the patient's serum potassium is normal or low, 1—1·5 ml potassium chloride injection, containing 1 gm in 5 ml (2·7—4·0 mEq) are added to each litre.

One litre of dialysate is infused at a time in most patients. Two-litre exchanges are more efficient but cause more pain and give a high incidence of respiratory complications. The infusion is made as rapidly as possible and the dialysate is allowed to dwell in the peritoneum for twenty minutes before being drained by siphonage into a 3-litre disposable plastic drainage bag, suspended below the patient's bed. The sequence is repeated as soon as drainage is complete, so that two exchanges are made each hour. The bag is emptied through its spigotted outlet into a measuring cylinder after each exchange. The input, output and progressive balance are charted (Fig. 3.8), so that a check can be kept to ensure that there is a negative balance at all times and fluid is not accumulating within the peritoneal cavity. If free drainage does not occur, the catheter should be

Acute Renal Failure

PERITONEAL DIALYSIS CHART	NAME ....
	DATE

INSTRUCTIONS	DIALYSATE
	ADDITIONS TO DIALYSATE
	VOLUME OF EXCHANGES
	DURATION OF EXCHANGES

TIME	INPUT				OUTPUT		BALANCE
	DIALYSATE	ADDITIONS	VOLUME GIVEN	PROGRESSIVE INPUT	VOLUME DRAINED	PROGRESSIVE DRAINAGE	

Fig. 3.8. Part of record chart for peritoneal dialysis.

flushed through, its position readjusted or, if necessary, it should be replaced. An important point to remember is that the dialysate containers hold more than one litre of fluid, and that the excess is variable. When a precise measure of dialysate input is necessary, as in infants, the container should be suspended from a spring balance, and the volume given determined by its change in weight.

Composition of Dialysate. The dialysate for routine use contains 1·36% dextrose. This is sufficiently hypertonic to plasma to ensure a modest negative water balance so that about two litres of fluid are removed from the patient in twenty-four hours of continuous dialysis. A solution containing 6·36% dextrose is also available but this is too hypertonic to be used alone for more than one or two exchanges, and then only for the relief of acute pulmonary oedema. For most overhydrated patients 500 ml of 1·36% solution should be infused concurrently to 500 ml of 6·36% solution. Even with this mixture, fluid can be removed from the circulation faster than it can diffuse into it from the interstitial fluid, and a careful watch should be kept for signs of hypovolaemia.

Most solutions have a sodium concentration of 141 mEq/1 but one with a concentration of 130 mEq/1 makes the control of hypertension easier, and also prevents the hypernatraemia which sometimes occurs in patients having hypertonic dialysis.

117

Peritonitis. Peritonitis developing as a complication of dialysis may produce some abdominal pain, but is often without symptoms or signs. It is indicated by turbidity of the dialysate and confirmed by finding pus cells on microscopy. There is no need to discontinue dialysis and it is treated by adding antibiotics to the dialysate. While awaiting the results of bacteriological culture, chloramphenicol 50 mg per litre or gentamicin 5 mg per litre are used. Most cases of peritonitis can be prevented by changing the catheter site routinely every three days, or earlier if there is any sign of local inflammation or leakage.

Duration of Dialysis. An initial period of thirty-six to forty-eight hours of continuous dialysis is usually needed to bring the uraemia under control and then about twelve hours each day will maintain a stable blood urea in most non-hypercatabolic patients. Between dialyses the catheter should be spigotted and the patient allowed to be up and about.

FURTHER READING

Merrill, J. P. (1971) in *Diseases of the Kidney*, edited by Strauss, M. B., and Welt, L. G., 2nd ed., p. 637, Churchill/Livingstone, London.
Muehrcke, R. C. (1969). *Acute Renal Failure: Diagnosis and Management*, Kimpton, London.
Schreiner, G. E. (1967) in *Renal Disease,* edited by D. A. K. Black, 2nd ed., p. 309, Blackwell, Oxford.

Chapter 4

Liver Disease and Intensive Care

IAIN M. MURRAY-LYON

INTRODUCTION

TRAUMA

FULMINANT HEPATIC FAILURE

CHRONIC HEPATIC FAILURE
　Bleeding Oesophageal Varices
　Ascites
　Hepatic Encephalopathy

SUPPURATIVE CHOLANGITIS

PATIENT DEVELOPING JAUNDICE IN HOSPITAL

INTRODUCTION

Although patients with liver disease make up a small fraction of the Intensive Care Unit population, they represent an important specialized group and there is evidence that their numbers are growing. As they often have complex metabolic problems and complications involving several systems, they are best cared for within the multidisciplinary framework of an intensive care

119

area. The increasing traffic congestion on the roads has brought with it a rising number of hepatic injuries as part of the spectrum of serious trauma. Fulminant hepatic failure is being forcibly drawn to medical and public attention by the continuing outbreaks of severe hepatitis in renal dialysis units. The annual death rate from cirrhosis in Europe is rising and many of these patients will first present with massive bleeding from oesophageal varices. Furthermore, patients with pre-existing chronic liver disease very readily become decompensated and develop hepatic encephalopathy or ascites in response to infection or trauma and this greatly modifies their medical management.

TRAUMA

Surgical Anatomy

The conventional description of the division of the liver into the left and the right lobe by the falciform ligament and ligamentum teres is misleading and inaccurate. The line of functional division lies to the right of the attachment of the falciform ligament and follows an imaginary line from the inferior vena cava obliquely across the upper surface of the liver to the gall bladder. These functional right and left lobes are supplied by the right and left hepatic arteries and branches of the portal vein on a fairly constant segmental basis, and are drained by hepatic veins which tend to lie between the segments. The bile ducts follow the course of the hepatic arteries and portal vein. There are few anastomoses between the vascular structures in the different segments and for this reason damage to a major segmental vessel will devitalize the whole segment, and liver injuries must always may be diminished by T tube decompression of the common

Type of Wound

Knife injuries produce clean incised wounds and carry a low mortality as they are rapidly diagnosed and treated. A major segmental vessel can, however, be severed requiring a segmental resection. Gun shot wounds and bursting injuries, usually due to road traffic accidents are more serious and there may be extensive liver damage with haemorrhage and bile leakage.

Diagnosis

There are no specific diagnostic features but hepatic trauma should always be suspected in accident cases as injuries are often multiple and sometimes the abdominal symptoms and signs may be delayed for some hours or even days. It is vital to remember that a head injury by itself rarely causes shock which should prompt a search for blood loss. The main complaint is of abdominal pain which may be worse on deep breathing and may radiate to one or other shoulder. The pain may be upper abdominal or widely spread. The physical findings are those of blood loss and local tenderness and rebound are often present. A subcapsular haematoma may be palpable.

Laboratory tests are of little help. The 4 quadrants of the abdomen should be tapped with a fine needle and this often yields blood or bile although a negative result does not exclude hepatic injury. More sophisticated procedures such as coeliac angiography and liver scintiscanning may be helpful in selective cases.

Management

Primary goals are haemostasis, removal of devitalized tissue, adequate drainage and measures to minimize late bleeding or bile leakage. Following initial resuscitation, operation is now regarded as an essential part of the management of liver injuries. Simple incised wounds may be sutured although debridement or segmental resection may be required if segmental vessels are damaged. Subcapsular haematomas should be incised and evacuated and the parenchymal tear repaired. More severe devitalizing injuries should be managed by debridement and simple drainage but in some cases partial hepatectomy will be needed. Packing of liver wounds has been largely abandoned because of the high risk of infection. The peritoneal cavity is invariably drained and bile leakage from lacerated liver may be diminished by T tube decompression of the common bile duct.

Post-operative Care of Liver Injuries and Hepatic Resections.
Careful management of fluid and electrolyte balance is

important as there may be large losses from drains and a common bile duct T-tube. After major hepatic resections there may be difficulty in maintaining the blood sugar and dextrose infusions will be needed; similarly infusions of albumin (25–75 g/day) may be required to keep up the serum level.

Rarely a severe coagulation defect develops post-operatively and vitamin K should be given routinely but fresh blood and fresh frozen plasma may also be needed. Delayed bleeding from the liver is most likely to occur when devitalized tissue remains or infection develops. Haemobilia is uncommon but may be massive and is usually due to a connection between the hepatic artery and a bile duct within an area of necrosis. Hepatic resection or ligation of the appropriate branch of the hepatic artery is often required.

Respiratory complications are common especially if there are fractured ribs or a thoracoabdominal surgical approach was used. Endotracheal intubation and assisted ventilation may be required.

Many surgeons recommend routine post-operative antibiotics especially if there is extensive hepatic injury or injury to other intra-abdominal organs.

FULMINANT HEPATIC FAILURE

This is the clinical syndrome associated with massive necrosis of liver cells or with sudden severe impairment of hepatic function. It is characterized by acute onset of progressive mental changes starting with confusion and rapidly advancing to stupor or coma. Jaundice appears and rapidly deepens, serum transaminases are markedly raised and the prothrombin time is prolonged. The whole illness from the first symptom till death may be a week or less but in some cases the course is more prolonged.

Aetiology

The cause in most cases is presumed to be due to viral hepatitis but drugs such as paracetamol and the monamine-oxidase inhibitors are also important. Hepatitis can occur as part of the illness caused by a number of viruses including these responsible for infective mononucleosis, cytomegalovirus disease and Herpes simplex but infectious (or short incubation) hepatitis and serum (or long incubation) hepatitis are far more common. It is probably impossible to distinguish between these two clinically and pathologically but there are epidemiological differences. Infective hepatitis is spread in an epidemic setting by the faecal-oral route, although sporadic cases can be transmitted parenterally like serum hepatitis by dirty needles or infected blood and blood products. There is now evidence that serum hepatitis can also be spread by the faecal-oral route. These illnesses are usually mild and self-limiting but occasional cases follow a fulminant course.

Australia-antigen (Hepatitis-associated antigen or Serum hepatitis antigen). This antigen was first detected in the serum of an Australian aborigine by Blumberg in 1965. Subsequent work has clearly associated it with the agent responsible for long incubation (serum) hepatitis but whether it is identical with the serum hepatitis virus awaits further study. The antigen can be detected by immunodiffusion or immunoelectrophoresis in the blood of a large proportion of early cases of long incubation hepatitis but it has not been detected in most closed outbreaks of infectious hepatitis. It is also found in a certain proportion of cases of some types of chronic liver disease including active chronic hepatitis and cryptogenic cirrhosis and in a small percentage (0·5—2·0%) of apparently normal people in whom carriage of the antigen is usually temporary. Certain other categories of patients, particularly those having multiple blood transfusions, also seem to have a higher than normal carriage rate with little disturbance in liver function and these include patients with leukaemia and chronic renal failure. Transfusion of Australia-antigen containing blood has been shown in many cases to be followed by hepatitis.

The patient who is Australia-antigen positive does represent a risk to other patients and staff and great care should be taken with venesection and other procedures in which blood may be spilt, and surgical gloves and gowns should be worn. This is particularly important in dealing with chronic haemodialysis patients. The patient should have his own cutlery and crockery and care must be taken with the disposal of excreta as the antigen has been detected in urine and stools. Regular screening of patients and staff in high risk areas for Australia-antigen should help to detect carriers and prevent spread and it seems likely that in the future all blood donors will be screened so as to minimize this important source of infection. Prophylactic gammaglobulin has not been shown to give full protection against infection with long incubation hepatitis although it is of value in preventing short incubation hepatitis.

Pathology

The liver is usually markedly reduced in size and the cut surface shows a mottled appearance with red areas of haemorrhage alternating with yellow patches of necrosis. In patients who have survived two weeks or more from the onset there may be nodules of regenerating tissue. Histologically, there is extensive loss of parenchymal cells and collapse of the reticulin framework with condensation of surviving bile ducts.

Clinical Syndrome

The neuropsychiatric changes are the most obvious clinically and the patient may present with a personality change, psychosis or the picture of meningo-encephalitis. Foetor hepaticus is common. Jaundice at this stage may be inconspicuous. Daily estimation of hepatic size is useful in patients with acute hepatitis and shrinking liver size is an ominous sign. There is progressive depression of brain stem function with increasing drowsiness leading to coma. Tendon reflexes become brisk and plantar responses extensor. Focal and generalized seizures often occur and terminally the cardiovascular and respiratory centres fail. The conscious level is usually graded according to the criteria of the Boston Fulminant Hepatic Failure Surveillance study:

Grade 0 — normal awareness
Grade I — mood change and confusion
Grade II — drowsiness
Grade III — stuporose
Grade IV — unrousable with minimal or no response to noxious stimuli.

The survival rate is 66% in those with Grade II encephalopathy but only 17% in those with Grade IV coma. The overall mortality in the first 318 patients reported from centres throughout the world to the Boston Survey was 82%.

Management

The object of treatment is to support life long enough until the damaging process is arrested and sufficient regeneration of the hepatic cells to maintain life occurs. Evidence of regeneration may be present histologically by about two weeks from the onset of the illness.

Encephalopathy. The main factor in the production of encephalopathy appears to be failure of the damaged liver to detoxicate substances absorbed into the blood following breakdown of nitrogenous materials in the colon, although electrolyte and acid base imbalance may also be important. Withdrawal of oral protein, emptying the bowel by enema and oral neomycin therapy (1 g six-hourly) to reduce the bacterial flora of the colon, are all important. Sedative drugs should be avoided if possible even if the patient is noisy, although small doses of phenobarbitone (30—60 mg) or diazepam (5—10 mg) may be needed.

Hypoglycaemia and Other Metabolic Changes. Careful monitoring of the blood chemistry is essential, for important metabolic changes occur in addition to the obvious disturbance in liver function. Profound hypoglycaemia should not be overlooked and the blood glucose should be measured every four hours. If hypoglycaemia develops massive amounts of glucose may be needed. It is important to remember that the flapping tremor and signs of a pyramidal lesion may be due to hypoglycaemia. Serum electrolytes need frequent estimation and supplementary potassium is almost always needed. Complex acid base changes occur. Initially, the patients often hyperventilate and develop a respiratory alkalosis, but later as a result of the massive liver damage lactic acid and other metabolites accumulate and lead to metabolic acidosis. Beneficial results may be achieved by intravenous bicarbonate infusion (500 ml 5%). Hypokalaemia may be associated with a metabolic alkalosis.

Coagulation Changes. Haemostasis is severly impaired in fulminant hepatic failure due to a combination of diminished synthesis of coagulation factors by the liver and intravascular coagulation. This is probably triggered off by contact of the blood with damaged liver cells and results in consumption of

125

platelets and clotting factors, thus throwing an extra strain on the already overtaxed production capacity of the liver for the proteins concerned with coagulation. The bleeding when it occurs is usually from the gastrointestinal tract often with skin purpura.

A central venous pressure line is valuable to detect blood volume depletion. This is usually due to bleeding which can be concealed in the retroperitoneal tissues and transfusion of fresh blood is desirable. The coagulation defect is monitored by daily prothrombin time and partial thromboplastin time, and an attempt may be made to stop further consumption of coagulation factors using continuous heparin infusion monitored by careful protamine titration. Between 20 and 30,000 units of heparin are usually required daily. This regime must be combined with infusion of 2–3 bottles of fresh frozen plasma daily to compensate for diminished hepatic synthesis of clotting factors.

Renal Failure. Renal failure is common in these patients and should be treated energetically, for a rising blood urea is one of the factors which seems to precipitate gastro-intestinal haemorrhage. The blood pressure should be maintained by transfusion and an adequate calorie intake in the form of intravenous hypertonic dextrose or dextrose by gastric tube is important, but care must be taken to avoid fluid overload. Urine flow should be maintained with intravenous 5% mannitol and frusemide, and peritoneal dialysis may be required.

Infection. A daily chest X-ray should be taken because of the high risk of aspiration and hypostatic pneumonia and early tracheostomy and assisted ventilation will often be needed and do not preclude eventual recovery. Indwelling catheters should be changed every 2–3 days and great care should be taken to avoid drip site sepsis. Barrier nursing to minimize cross infection is also worthwhile.

OTHER MEASURES: In many patients, despite careful nursing and medical care, the clinical course is inexorably downhill and other life saving forms of treatment need to be considered. In some of these patients super-imposed acute pancreatitis may be responsible for the deterioration.

Corticosteroid Drugs. These are often given although there is no evidence of their efficacy in this context. Their possible beneficial effects have to be balanced against the increased risk of infection and gastro-intestinal haemorrhage which often accompanies their use.

Exchange Transfusion. About 50—60% of patients with fulminant hepatic failure will show temporary improvement following exchange transfusion. The recommended technique if to exchange 1½—2 times the calculated blood volume over 2—3 hours, blood being simultaneously infused through a vein and withdrawn from an artery. In Australia-antigen positive patients there is considerable risk to staff. Fresh blood is desirable and care should be taken to warm the blood before transfusion and to balance the volumes exchanged. Arterial blood gases and plasma electrolytes should be carefully monitored as these may become markedly disturbed particularly when using stored blood. Intravenous calcium gluconate (10 ml 10% solution) should be given after every second bottle of citrated blood.

The initial enthusiasm for the procedure has waned recently and a controlled trial in patients failed to show any benefit.

Extracorporeal Liver Perfusion and Other Methods of Temporary Liver Support. Livers from several animal species and human cadavers have been used. After careful hepatectomy the isolated liver is set up in a perfusion circuit and perfused with fresh blood compatible with the patient. The patient's circulation is then connected. Animal livers will function for up to 8 hours and human livers for up to 35 hours, bile is produced and bilirubin and ammonia are extracted from the patient's blood. Although temporary improvement with return of consciousness has been reported, the benefits are short lasting and repeated periods of perfusion with fresh livers are usually required. Only a handful of patients have survived and the complexities of the procedure confine its use to specialized centres.

Cross-circulation between a patient with fulminant hepatic failure and a person without liver disease or a non-human primate has been tried on a number of occasions. The procedure is not without risk to the donor and it is obviously applicable only when there is no question of a viral aetiology of the massive hepatic necrosis.

Haemodialysis and peritoneal dialysis to remove ammonia and other dialysable compounds have met with almost uniform failure but the development of newer membranes with different physical properties may improve the prospects.

Plasmaphoresis in which the patient's plasma is separated and discarded and the red cells and platelets are resuspended in fresh frozen plasma and reinfused has sometimes proved effective at reversing encephalopathy and is worthy of further trial.

Transplantation of the liver offers some hope of recovery but the operation on an Australia-antigen positive recipient carries a considerable risk to staff and it is usually difficult to find a suitable donor in the short space of time available.

MANAGEMENT OF CHRONIC LIVER FAILURE

Patients with cirrhosis may first present with bleeding oesophageal varices, ascites or encephalopathy but they are not immune from other medical and surgical conditions and previously unsuspected cirrhosis may be discovered in hospital when ascites or hepatic encephalopathy develop unexpectedly following infection, a myocardial infarction or operation. Careful physical examination will often reveal spider naevi, palmar erythema, splenomegaly or other stigmata of chronic liver disease but in some cases there may be no specific signs. The development of a malignant hepatoma is a further cause for deterioration of liver function in cirrhosis.

General Management

The factor precipitating decompensation should be corrected as quickly as possible. The cirrhotic patient is particularly liable to develop a septicaemia and frequent blood cultures should be taken if this is suspected and broad spectrum antibiotics are often started empirically. Vitamins (including vitamin K) should be given parenterally with a high calorie intake (2500 calories daily). Protein intake should be 50—70 g daily unless there are signs of hepatic encephalopathy. Parenteral feeding may be required in some cases but care should be taken to control the sodium intake which should be restricted in known cirrhotics to 50 mEq daily and less if ascites is present. Care should be taken with intravenous amino acid preparations as these may precipitate encephalopathy.

Patients with liver disease are very sensitive to the effects of sedatives and analgesics particularly paraldehyde and morphine and their use should be minimized. If sedation is required small doses of phenobarbitone (6—120 mg) or diazepam (5—10 mg) may be tried.

Bleeding Oesophageal Varices

Haemorrhage from oesophageal varices is one of the most formidable emergencies in medicine. It accounts for around 3 per cent of patients presenting with a haematemesis and carries a mortality of between 40 and 70 per cent. These patients die from a combination of blood loss and liver failure which is exacerbated by the drop in blood flow and hepatic anoxia which results from the haemorrhage. In addition, the blood in the lumen of the gut acts as a large protein load and contributes to the development of hepatic encephalopathy. The aim of treatment must be to stop haemorrhage by the fastest and simplest method available.

Diagnosis. Many of the patients will be known to have cirrhosis or will have classical signs of chronic hepatic parenchymal disease such as spider naevi, palmar erythema and leukonychia. These will be absent in the rare group of patients with portal hypertension due to extrahepatic block. Splenomegaly is usual but the spleen may sometimes become impalpable after the onset of haemorrhage.

It is important to determine the site of bleeding as cirrhotic patients have an increased incidence of peptic ulcer and the alcoholic may have gastric erosions. A barium swallow and meal

129

should, therefore, be performed; where there is doubt about the site of bleeding, endoscopic examination of the oesophagus, stomach and duodenum may be required. The development of fibreoptic instruments has now made this a simple procedure. Control of bleeding by the Sengstaken tube is a useful confirmatory test.

Treatment

Blood transfusion will be required in most cases and it is essential to maintain good hepatic circulation and prevent further impairment of liver cell function. Sodium should be given sparingly because it is likely to result in ascites and the intravenous infusion should be kept open with 5% dextrose.

The bowels should be emptied by purgation with oral magnesium sulphate (10 ml of 10% solution) every 4—6 hours and by enemata twice daily. Neomycin is given by mouth as elixir (1 g six-hourly) to decrease bacterial breakdown of protein in the bowel and dietary protein is omitted.

If the bleeding continues or recurs other measures are required (Fig. 4.1).

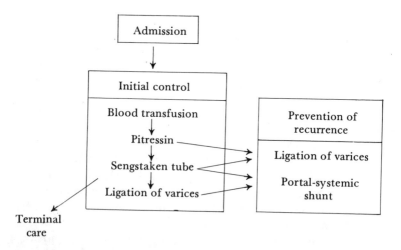

Fig. 4.1. Management of the patient with bleeding oesophageal varices (after Williams and Dawson, 1968).

130

Vasopressin. Vasopressin lowers the portal venous pressure by constricting the splanchnic arterioles and limiting the inflow of blood to the gut. It is given as an intravenous infusion of 20 units in 100 ml of 5% dextrose over 20 minutes. (Ensure that the aqueous preparation is used — it should be kept in the refrigerator.) It produces arteriolar constriction with pallor of the skin and its use is contraindicated with patients with ischaemic heart disease because of its action on the coronary arteries. Intestinal colic usually accompanies its use and this helps to empty the bowel. The effects last for an hour or more and the dose can be repeated after 2—4 hours although further doses tend to be less effective. The bleeding can be controlled initially in 70—80% of cases although it usually restarts later.

Sengstaken Tube. If vasopressin is ineffective or the bleeding restarts the Sengstaken tube is the next line of defence. It is a triple lumen tube combining gastric and oesophageal balloons and a nasogastric suction tube (Fig. 4.2). Unless the patient is co-operative and able to swallow it is difficult to position a soft rubber tube and models made in a stiffer material are preferable.* Before use the balloons should be checked for patency and leaks and the ends of the 3 lumens are clearly labelled. The throat should be anaesthetized with topical anaesthetic and the tube lubricated with local anaesthetic jelly. When the tube has passed well into the stomach, the gastric balloon is filled with 80—100 ml of radio-opaque solution and the end of that lumen is clamped with forceps. The tube is pulled up so that the gastric balloon lodges at the cardio-oesophageal junction and compresses gastric varices. Its use is contraindicated in patients with a hiatus hernia. The position is maintained by taping the tube firmly to the face and traction over a pulley wheel is seldom required. The oesophageal balloon is now inflated with air to 30—35 mm Hg using a sphygmomanometer and a three-way tap arrangement to check and maintain the pressure. The third lumen is used for gastric suction and administering drugs. If the bleeding was from oesophageal varices it will now usually be controlled. The position of the tube should be checked radio-logically with a portable film. If the tube becomes dislodged,

*Obtainable from J. G. Franklin & Sons, Cressex, High Wycombe, Bucks.

131

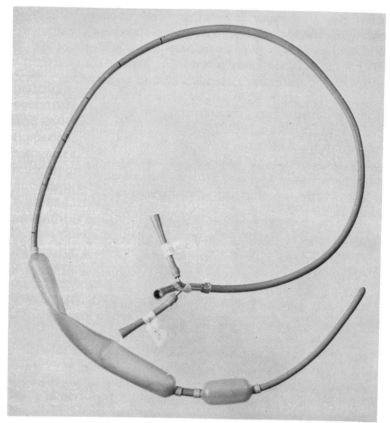

Fig. 4.2. Sengstaken triple lumen tube.

the oesophageal balloon may obstruct the larynx and the nurses must be instructed to deflate the balloons immediately. The tube may be left in position for 24—36 hours but the oesophageal balloon should be let down for a few minutes every hour and the balloon pressure checked regularly. Repeated pharyngeal suction will be required.

The use of the tube is commonly associated with the development of chest infection and oesophageal ulceration which may predispose to further haemorrhage.

Bleeding often restarts soon after removal of the tube and consideration should be given early to the timing of an operation

132

if this is planned. It is then best to leave the tube in situ till the patient is taken to the operating theatre.

Other Non-surgical Techniques. Gastric cooling is well tolerated and probably as effective as the two previous methods but it requires specialized apparatus and is attended by a high risk of pulmonary complications.

Injection of sclerosing solutions into and around the varices at oesophagoscopy has been tried by several workers with variable results.

Continuous infusion of vasopressin into the superior mesenteric artery through a catheter sited by the percutaneous Seldinger approach through the femoral artery has been reported to reduce portal venous pressure and control bleeding. However the technique is attended by a high incidence of complications and control of haemorrhage is usually only temporary.

Emergency Surgery

Whether or not the bleeding has been completely controlled by the Sengstaken tube, consideration should be given to surgery because of the limited time the tube may be left in position and the high risk of recurrent bleeding after its removal. In patients with jaundice, ascites, encephalopathy and gross prolongation of the prothrombin time before the haemorrhage, the bleeding is part of the picture of terminal liver failure and surgery is seldom indicated. However, in others, an attempt should be made to control the bleeding surgically. As each haemorrhage is accompanied by further deterioration in liver function and the chances of a successful outcome diminish, operation should be done early rather than late.

Surgical Ligation of Varices. This is the easiest and quickest procedure. A left thoracotomy is used to obtain surgical access to the lower oesophagus which is mobilized. In the Boerema–Crile operation the lower oesophageal lumen is entered via a longitudinal incision and the varices are under-run with a continuous catgut suture. In the Milnes–Walker operation the

133

muscle of the lower oesophagus is divided longitudinally down to the mucosa and the oesophageal mucosal tube is divided transversely and resutured. This suture and the healing process in the mucosal layer occludes the varices.

After this operation oral fluids are prohibited for five days and a gastrografin swallow is then performed to exclude an anastomotic leak. It is usual for these patients to have one to two weeks post-operative pyrexia, possibly due to thombosis of the varices.

A more extensive thoraco-abdominal attack on the collaterals (porta-azygos disconnection is also sometimes performed. The immediate results of these operations depend on the hepatic reserves. Many patients die with post-operative hepatic or renal failure even though the bleeding does not recur.

Other Methods. The mortality of an emergency portacaval shunt is 40—50 per cent and this excludes the operation from consideration except in patients with excellent liver function in whom good results may be obtained.

The thoracic duct in patients with cirrhosis is often distended and contains lymph under pressure. Cannulation of the duct and drainage of lymph may result in reduction in portal pressure but the procedure has not proved successful in controlling variceal bleeding in most cases.

Prevention of Further Bleeding. Bleeding from oesophageal varices usually recurs within weeks or months and this is true even after the varices have been ligated although some patients remain well for long periods. All patients should, therefore, be assessed for definitive surgery. The most successful operation is a portacaval shunt. Ideally, the patient should be less than 50 years old, without jaundice, with a serum albumin greater than 3 g/100 ml and have no evidence of hepatic encephalopathy even during haemorrhage. However, many less favourable patients will benefit from the operation although the risk of post-operative liver failure and hepatic encephalopathy will be greater. In patients with an extrahepatic portal vein block, in whom liver function is usually well preserved, a splenorenal or mesenteric-caval shunt is often the only type of operation possible.

Results

The mortality in the first year after bleeding from oesophageal varices varies from 33—90 per cent, the wide variation being a reflection of the severity of the underlying liver disease in the series of patients studied. A high mortality can be expected in any form of surgery in patients with liver failure and even in patients with good liver function the operative mortality following ligation of varices is 30—50 per cent. Many of these patients will be suitable for subsequent portacaval anastomosis and there is no doubt that a successful shunt can prevent further haemorrhage. However, there is a 20 per cent incidence of overt hepatic encephalopathy which may be severely disabling in some patients. Although spleno-renal anastomosis has a lower incidence of hepatic encephalopathy it is less effective at preventing a further haemorrhage and there is a higher risk of the shunt clotting. The five-year survival following an elective portacaval anastomosis lies between 30 and 55 per cent. There is at present no evidence that a prophylactic portacaval shunt in patients with oesophageal varices who have not bled prolongs survival, although the incidence of bleeding is decreased.

Ascites

The two most important factors in the development of ascites in liver disease are a low serum albumin concentration and increased portal venous pressure. More fluid enters the peritoneal cavity than leaves it. For reasons which are incompletely understood, secondary hyperaldosteronism develops and may be important in perpetuating the ascites. The effect of the high levels of circulating aldosterone is to increase renal tubular absorption of sodium so that urinary sodium excretion is often less than 5 mEq daily. Despite this, the serum sodium concentration is often deceptively low for the total body sodium content is greatly increased. The serum potassium concentration is usually normal or slightly depressed although the total body exchangeable potassium is decreased because of increased urinary losses.

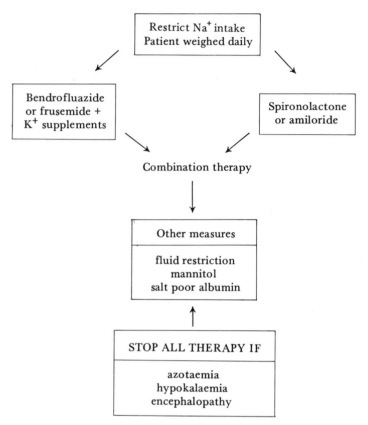

Fig. 4.3. Treatment of ascites.

Treatment. The first essential is to control sodium intake both in the diet and in intravenous fluids (Fig. 4.3). Many parenteral fluid regimes contain large amounts of sodium and during treatment of the ascites total daily sodium intake should be reduced to a maximum of 22 mEq (0·5 g). Abdominal paracentesis should be avoided as this removes large quantities of protein and increases the risk of peritoneal infection, but it is wise to perform one diagnostic aspiration with a fine needle to obtain fluid for culture and cytological examination. Diuretics will usually be required and the dosage should be controlled according to the patient's daily weight loss. The aim is to reduce the body weight by about 800 g daily as it has been shown that this represents the maximal rate of absorption of ascites. Greater losses occur at the expense of the plasma volume and tend to result in deterioration in renal function. The diuretics must then be stopped. It is wise to start with a small dose of diuretic and increase this slowly. Suitable starting regimes are either bendrofluazide 10—20 mg daily or frusemide 40 mg—80 mg daily. Generous potassium chloride supplementation should be given (100—150 mEq/day as Slow-K or Kloref) and a careful check kept on the plasma potassium concentration. If these drugs do not result in a satisfactory diuresis it is helpful to add the aldosterone antagonist spironolactone (25—50 mg q.i.d.). Recently, this drug has also been shown to be effective when used alone. The dose is gradually increased up to a maximum of 1 g daily until the ratio of the urinary excretion of sodium and potassium is greater than 1. Oral potassium supplements are not usually required, either with spironolactone or with the recently introduced potassium sparing diuretic amiloride which is given in a dose of up to 5 mg q.d.s. The powerful diuretic ethacrynic acid is seldom required and its use is often associated with the development of serious electrolyte disturbance. In resistant cases infusion of mannitol or salt-free albumin (25—50 g per day) may sometimes be helpful in starting a diuresis.

Results and Complications. The combination of strict sodium restriction and careful diuretic therapy usually results in control of ascites. Hypokolaemia should be carefully looked for and treated vigorously. Hypovolaemia due to excessive fluid loss leads to azotaemia and diuretic therapy should be temporarily suspended if the blood urea starts to rise significantly. Hyponatraemia reflects urinary excretion of sodium in excess of water and in a critically ill patient may also be due to passage of sodium into the cells. Fluid restriction to 500 ml daily or intravenous mannitol (250 ml 10%) should be tried. Sodium supplementation is seldom effective and results in further increase in fluid retention. However, occasionally following prolonged diuretic therapy after clearance of oedema and ascites, patients can become sodium depleted and in these rare circumstances sodium supplements are urgently required. Hepatic encephalopathy may be precipitated or exacerbated by diuretic therapy which is then best temporarily suspended.

Hepatic Encephalopathy

The clinical picture is complex and variable. There is usually a
disturbance of consciousness ranging from slight drowsiness to
coma. Mood fluctuates from apathy to wild excitement and
frankly psychotic symptoms may dominate the picture. One of
the earliest psychiatric changes is an inability to copy a five-
pointed star (constructional apaxia). The most characteristic
although not specific neurological sign is the flapping tremor of
the outstretched hand. Disorder of the pyramidal system is
common with brisk reflexes, ankle clonus and extensor plantar
responses, but cerebellar and extrapyramidal signs may also
appear. In severe cases, focal and generalized convulsions may
occur. Patients with hepatic encephalopathy are suffering from
cerebral intoxication by intestinal contents which have not been
mtabolized by the liver. The nature of the toxins is still specula-
tive but ammonia is probably important.

Treatment. The treatment is based on preventing further formation of nitrogenous products in the bowel by bacteria and
correcting any precipitating factors such as infection, sedative
drugs, electrolyte imbalance or gastro-intestinal haemorrhage
(Fig. 4.4).
Dietary protein is stopped and an adequate calorie intake
ensured (2500 calories per day). This is usually given as 10—20%
glucose by large intravenous cannula unless the patient is able to
take food by mouth. During recovery protein is gradually re-
introduced in 10—20 g increments. The bowels are evacuated
with enemas and oral magnesium sulphate (10 ml 10% solution,
2—3 times daily) to ensure a daily bowel motion. Broad
spectrum antibiotics are given orally and neomycin 1 g 6-hourly
is usually chosen. Lactulose, which is a non-absorbable disac-
charide, is also useful. It is broken down in the colon by
bacteria to organic acids and its beneficial action is probably
due to trapping of ammonia in the acidified bowel contents. It
is useful to start with 25—50 ml of syrup t.d.s. and to adjust the
dose to obtain 2—3 semi-fluid stools daily. Some patients
require 150 ml daily or more whereas others get troublesome
diarrhoea with under 100 ml.

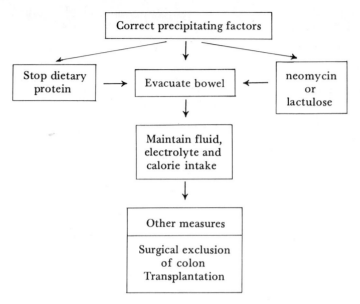

Fig. 4.4. Treatment of hepatic encephalopathy.

Some patients with chronic disabling hepatic encephalopathy may be resistant to the above therapy and for long-term management consideration should be given to surgical exclusion of the colon and transplantation of the liver.

SUPPURATIVE CHOLANGITIS

Cholangitis is rare unless there is biliary obstruction, usually due to gall stones, which may be visible on plain radiographs of the abdomen. It is characterized by jaundice, fever and upper abdominal pain. Gram negative organisms are usually responsible. It is a serious condition and oliguric renal failure is a common complication for conjugated bilirubin sensitizes the kidney to ischaemic damage. A considerable measure of protection is afforded by mannitol infusions. Some patients rapidly deteriorate and die of septicaemia despite all resuscitative efforts.

Management

Blood cultures are taken and parenteral antibiotics started. Penetration into the obstructed biliary tree may be severely

139

limited but ampicillin (1 g six-hourly) or rifamide (150 mg 8-hourly) are the most likely to be effective. Vitamin K is given intramuscularly.

Regular measurement of blood pressure and central venous pressure should be made and hourly urine output charted. Large volumes of colloid may be required to maintain the circulating blood volume in patients with Gram negative septicaemia. Mannitol should be given if necessary to maintain urine flow above 1 ml/min.

If there is no definite improvement within 24—48 hours, emergency surgery to establish biliary drainage should be undertaken. Percutaneous transhepatic cholangiography should be performed immediately prior to surgery to demonstrate the anatomical site of the obstruction, and aspirated bile is sent for culture. If the obstruction is due to stones in the common bile duct, T-tube drainage may be life-saving. Definitive removal of stones and the gall bladder may be done at a later date.

Prophylactic mannitol should be given intravenously before and after operation to minimize the risk of post-operative renal failure. A suitable regime is to infuse 500 ml 10% mannitol beginning one hour before the operation. In the post-operative period, sufficient 5% mannitol is given to maintain the urine flow above 1 ml per minute for 48 hours. This usually requires around 500 ml mannitol in each 24-hour period.

PATIENTS DEVELOPING JAUNDICE IN HOSPITAL

Seriously ill patients may become jaundiced during their stay in hospital. Although there are many possible mechanisms and it may be difficult to define the precise cause in the individual case, particular attention should be paid to the anaesthetic, drug and blood pressure records, operative procedures and blood transfusion.

Pre-existing Chronic Liver Disease

The patient with cirrhosis tolerates surgery and infection badly and these may be followed by decompensation of the liver disease and development of jaundice, ascites or portal systemic encephalopathy.

Blood Transfusion

About 10% of the erythrocytes in 14-day-old acid-citrate dextrose blood are probably destroyed by the reticulo-endothelial system in the first 24 hours after transfusion. 500 ml blood which contains approximately 70 g haemoglobin therefore liberates about 7 g haemoglobin. This will be broken down to 250 mg bilirubin which is equivalent to the total normal daily bilirubin production. Thus when many pints of blood are transfused a greatly increased load of bilirubin will be presented to the liver for conjugation and excretion and a similar load will result from extensive tissue haematomata and pulmonary infarcts. It is well recognized that this haemolysis results in mild transient jaundice 24–48 hours after transfusion and although the bilirubin is predominantly unconjugated, a definite increase in the conjugated fraction may also occur. Unless there is coexistent liver disease, the total plasma bilirubin seldom exceeds 5 mg/100 ml because of the great capacity of the liver to handle pigment.

Virus Infection

Both the virus of serum hepatitis and cytomegalovirus are transmitted in blood although infections may also be contracted by other routes.

Serum Hepatitis. Recipients of Australia-antigen containing blood often develop hepatitis and Australia-antigen may be detected in their serum. The incubation period is variable but may be as short as two weeks or as long as 16 weeks. The liver is usually tender and enlarged and the spleen may be palpable. A rash and arthropathy occurs in a small proportion of cases. Liver function tests in addition to the increase in conjugated plasma bilirubin show a striking rise in serum aspartate transaminase. Recovery usually occurs over 4–6 weeks but occasional cases progress to fulminant hepatic failure (see above). No specific treatment is required.

Cytomegalovirus Hepatitis. Usually follows 2–4 weeks after transfusion of fresh blood but stored blood has also been

141

implicated. The illness is similar to infective mononucleosis but the Paul Bunnell test is consistently negative. Patients have fever, hepatomegaly and sometimes splenomegaly and a rash. The blood picture often shows atypical mononuclear cells. Liver function tests usually show a mixed cholestatic-hepatitic picture with marked elevation of the serum alkaline phosphatase and transaminases. Part of the increase in the plasma bilirubin may be in the unconjugated fraction as there is sometimes significant haemolysis. A rising titre of complement fixing antibodies to cytomegalovirus and isolation of the virus from a fresh specimen of urine are useful diagnostic tests. The illness is usually self-limiting.

Bacterial Infection

Jaundice may be due to extrahepatic bacterial infection. Septicaemia due to certain organisms such as *Cl. welchii* and *Str. pyogenes* may cause severe haemolysis, and other infections, often associated with bacteriaemia, may cause poorly understood hepatocellular dysfunction. This is seen particularly in children with *E. coli* pyelonephritis and in adults with serious infections with *pneumococci, staphylcocci* or *streptococci.* The serum bilirubin may rise to 15 mg/100 ml or more and the alkaline phosphatase is also often raised. Liver biopsy usually shows little change apart from cholestasis. Treatment of the underlying infection is followed by recovery.

Anaesthetic Agents

Jaundice has been occasionally recorded following most anaesthetic agents but recently halothane has fallen under suspicion. It seems likely but not certain that halothane is responsible for post-operative hepatitis in a very small percentage of patients, particularly those having multiple exposures. The reaction is probably a hypersensitivity phenomenon. Seven to 14 days following the first exposure there is unexplained fever and malaise and after re-exposure the rise in temperature is noted earlier. Jaundice appears rapidly after the fever 10—28 days after a single exposure but 3—17 days after multiple anaesthetics. This delay is useful in excluding other causes of post-operative icterus such as transfusion reactions, shock and benign post-operative cholestasis which occur earlier. Hepatomegaly and splenomegaly are rare. Liver function tests show a variable rise in bilirubin and very high serum transaminase. The alkaline phosphatase may occasionally be elevated. Positive mitochondrial antibodies have been found transiently in some patients. Tests for Australia-antigen are negative. Although the reported mortality from fulminant hepatic failure is 70—90% there are probably many minor and unrecognized cases, and clinicians must be alert to the significance of delayed post-operative fever and care must be taken to look for evidence of hypersensitivity before giving repeat halothane anaesthetics.

Other Drugs

Many drugs can cause jaundice by one of a variety of mechanisms. Direct hepatic toxicity is the most serious complication of paracetamol overdose and occurs in most patients taking more than 15 g. Some of these patients die with fulminant hepatic failure. Tetracycline may cause acute hepatic failure when given intravenously in large doses (2—6 g daily) especially during pregnancy. A hepatitis-like hypersensitivity reaction with a mortality of around 20% can follow mono-aminoxidase inhibitors, isoniazid and methyl dopa. A mixed cholestasis-hepatitis picture is produced in susceptible patients by phenothiazines, particularly chlorpromazine (Largactil), chlordiazepoxide (Librium), the tricyclic antidepressants and many other drugs, including sulphonamides and the popular combination with trimethoprin (Septrin, Bactrim). Pure cholestasis accompanies use of anabolic and androgenic steroids such as norethandrolone and methyltestosterone and the oral contraceptives containing oestrogen.

In all cases of jaundice a careful drug history should be taken and the current therapy list carefully scrutinized.

Circulatory Failure

The liver cells are particularly susceptible to anoxaemic damage and marked centrilobular necrosis may follow both severe congestive cardiac failure and peripheral circulatory failure with low blood pressure. In heart failure overt jaundice is rare, although in severe cases the serum bilirubin may be above 15 mg/ 100 ml. There is a moderate rise in serum transaminases but the alkaline phosphatase is usually normal. In shock, particularly if prolonged for more than a few hours, there may be severe hepatic damage with the clinical picture of fulminant hepatic failure in some cases.

Surgery

Minor disturbances in liver function often follow surgical procedures but overt jaundice beginning immediately after abdominal surgery may be due to trauma to the bile duct or rarely pancreatitis. Biliary obstruction is accompanied by marked elevation in serum alkaline phosphatase, but little change in transaminases. If the jaundice persists percutaneous transhepatic cholangiography should be done to locate the site of the obstruction immediately prior to reconstructive surgery.

Obstructive jaundice may also occur 1—4 days after surgery due to intrahepatic cholestasis. This is a poorly explained and self-limiting syndrome occurring particularly after major surgery with prolonged anaesthesia, periods of hypotension and multiple blood transfusion. Liver biopsy has shown little abnormality apart from cholestasis in most cases. The jaundice may persist for up to a month. This diagnosis should always be considered in the post-operative patient with deep jaundice, as surgical intervention is contra-indicated.

Cardiac Surgery. Jaundice seems particularly likely to follow major cardiac surgery such as double or triple valve replacement. Many factors probably play a part including the large volume of blood transfused with the increased risk of infection, hypotension and hypothermia during the operation and mechanical damage to blood by the heart/lung machine and the prosthetic valves.

FURTHER READING

Dawson, J. L. (1970). Recent advances in jaundice — surgical aspects, *British Medical Journal*, 1, 228.

Kantrowitz, P. A., Jones, W. A., Greenberger, N. J. and Isselbacher, K. J. (1967). Severe postoperative hyperbilirubinaemia simulating obstructive jaundice, *New England Journal of Medicine*, 276, 591.

Little, J. M. (1971). *The Management of Liver Injuries*, E. & S. Livingstone, Edinburgh & London.

Sherlock, S. (1968). *Diseases of the Liver and Biliary System*, 4th ed., Blackwell, Oxford & Edinburgh.

Shulman, N. R. (1970). Hepatitis-associated antigen, *American Journal of Medicine*, 49, 669.

Williams, R. (1971). Treatment of fulminant hepatic failure, *British Medical Journal*, 1, 213.

Williams, R. and Dawson, J. L. (1968). Management of bleeding oesophageal varices, *British Medical Journal*, 1, 35.

Chapter 5

Diabetic Coma and Some Other Endocrine Emergencies

JOANNA SHELDON

INTRODUCTION

SEVERE DIABETIC KETO-ACIDOSIS

DIABETIC COMA WITHOUT KETO-ACIDOSIS. (HYPEROSMOLAR COMA)

LACTIC ACIDOSIS

HYPOGLYCAEMIA

THYROID CRISIS

ACUTE ADRENAL INSUFFICIENCY

146

SECONDARY HYPOADRENALISM

MYXOEDEMA COMA

HYPERCALCAEMIC CRISIS

ACUTE HYPOCALCAEMIA

INTRODUCTION

Emergencies in patients with endocrine diseases are frequently preventable, arising often through sloth in diagnosis, and sometimes through inappropriate treatment. Recognition of the early symptoms and signs of these conditions is essential in order to prevent the final nose-dive into metabolic disaster. Emphasis in this chapter is therefore on diagnosis and early treatment, though diabetic coma is dealt with in greater detail, being a relatively common condition. It is not intended to discuss at length the relative merits of various different therapeutic regimes that have been adopted in these conditions, but rather to provide a regime of known efficacy and safety for each condition. Dosages apply to the average adult (70 kg), and may need modification to suit the individual.

Many patients with metabolic disturbances are drowsy or unconscious on admission. Hence their initial management may include establishing a satisfactory airway, assisting ventilation, supporting the circulation, and emptying the stomach to avoid aspiration of its contents. Central venous pressure monitoring may be important to prevent fluid overload during treatment, and careful recording of blood pressure, pulse and respiration rates, fluid intake and output, laboratory findings and treatment is essential. These conditions are not static, and if treatment is to be effective the changing situation requires frequent appraisal.

SEVERE DIABETIC KETO-ACIDOSIS

The term diabetic precoma refers to a patient who is conscious, but drowsy from severe diabetic keto-acidosis, and coma to one

147

who is unconscious. In spite of advances in the management of these conditions the mortality is usually around 5–10%, and is much higher in patients over 60. Mortality correlates more closely with age, the depth of coma and the presence of associated non-diabetic illness than with other features of the disease. Urgent treatment is essential, and continued vigilance is required until recovery is complete, so these patients should be nursed whenever possible in an Intensive Therapy Unit.

Pathophysiology of Diabetic Coma

The symptoms and signs of severe diabetic ketosis arise from lack of insulin (Fig. 5.1).

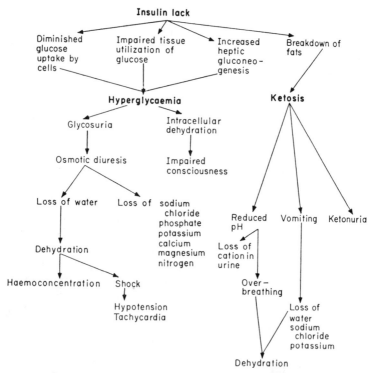

Fig. 5.1. Physiological disturbances in diabetic ketoacidosis. Reproduced from *Clinical Diabetes and its Biochemical Basis* ed. Oakley, Pyke and Taylor, Blackwell Scientific Publications 1968.

Lack of insulin diminishes transport of glucose into cells, as well as reducing intracellular utilization of glucose, both in glycolysis and in the synthesis of glycogen. In addition gluconeogenesis from precursors such as pyruvate and amino acids is increased. Hyperglycaemia is the result. Hyperglycaemia raises the osmotic pressure of the extracellular fluid, resulting in withdrawal of water from the cells, with intracellular dehydration, which may contribute to the loss of consciousness. In spite of this however, the osmolar concentration of the extracellular fluid, and of the glomerular filtrate, remains high. Isosmotic reabsorption of water from the proximal renal tubule is therefore restricted, and the distal tubule is presented with an excessive volume of fluid. The capacity for distal tubular reabsorption of water is exceeded, and there is an osmotic diuresis, with loss of electrolytes as well as water.

Insulin lack also increases the release of fatty acids from adipose tissue, and reduces the rate of fat synthesis. Lipolysis is accentuated by elevated levels of hydrocortisone, glucagon, growth hormone and adrenaline. One reason for the reduced fat synthesis is that glucose is the major source of carbon for fat synthesis, so that where glucose utilization is impaired, so is fat synthesis. Thus increased amounts of fatty acids pass to the liver for conversion to ketones (acetoacetate and hydroxybutyrate). Some of the acetoacetate is degraded to acetone. Keto-acidosis develops when the rate of production of ketones exceeds the rate of their utilization.

The acidosis is initially compensated by various buffer systems shown below, in which HK represents keto-acids.

$$HK + NaHCO_3 \rightarrow NaK + H_2CO_3 \rightarrow H_2O + CO_2$$

The bicarbonate buffer system increases production of carbonic acid from keto-acids and bicarbonate, and the rise in pCO_2 and fall in pH stimulates the respiratory centre. This causes the deep, rapid breathing (Kussmaul respiration) which helps to eliminate carbonic acid. It also contributes further to water loss.

The renal response to acidosis includes the almost complete reabsorption of bicarbonate, with replacement of urinary bicarbonate by anions of keto-acids combined with sodium. Keto-acids are also buffered by the urinary phosphate, with loss of sodium salts of keto-acids and sodium dihydrogen phospate:

$$HK + Na_2HPO_4 \rightarrow NaK + NaH_2PO_4$$

Increased rate of ammonia formation, with increased loss of urinary ammonium also helps to get rid of excess hydrogen ions. Finally the distal tubular exchange mechanism promotes hydrogen ion loss, while helping to limit sodium loss.

Vomiting contributes to the water and salt loss, and balance studies have shown that during the development of diabetic coma in an adult, about 6 litres of water may be lost, together with about 500 mEq of sodium, some 400 mEq of chloride and 200–350 mEq of potassium (Table I).

TABLE I. Losses in the development of diabetic coma

WATER	$\simeq$ 6 L
SODIUM	$\simeq$ 500 mEq
CHLORIDE	$\simeq$ 400 mEq
POTASSIUM	$\simeq$ 200–350 mEq

Clinical Features of Severe Diabetic Ketosis. A period of polyuria and polydipsia precedes the development of drowsiness in severe diabetic keto-acidosis. Weight loss is usually considerable and the patient has almost always been vomiting. These symptoms usually progress over a few days, or weeks, though occasionally, in young, established diabetics who miss a dose of insulin, the sequence of events may be so rapid that coma develops within a matter of hours. Abdominal pain, which can be so severe as to mimic an acute abdominal emergency, is not an uncommon manifestation of severe diabetic ketosis, particularly in the young.

The signs of severe diabetic keto-acidosis are characteristic. The patient is drowsy or unconscious, and *is almost always profoundly dehydrated*, often with a shrunken looking tongue. Breathing is usually rapid and deep, and the breath smells of acetone. Hypotension and tachycardia are usual and hypothermia may occur, even in the presence of infection. There may be gastric dilatation producing a succussion splash.

Heavy glycosuria and ketonuria are almost invariable, the very rare exceptions being patients with severe renal disease with a raised threshold for glucose and ketones. The blood sugar is always raised, and usually exceeds 500 mg per 100 ml.

Differential Diagnosis. In spite of this characteristic clinical picture misdiagnoses occur. Nausea and vomiting may be attributed to gastroenteritis, and overbreathing to pneumonia. Unconsciousness may be thought to result from a cerebrovascular accident, particularly in cases of aketotic coma (see p. 161), where, because of lack of acidosis there is no hyperventilation, and no smell of acetone on the breath. Uraemia and salicylism may both be accompanied by unconsciousness and overbreathing, and may at first be difficult to distinguish from diabetic coma if a history is not available. The severely uraemic patient will however usually be anaemic, and the blood urea will be higher than in diabetic coma, though in the latter it is commonly raised up to 100 mg per 100 ml as a result of dehydration. The patient with salicylate intoxication is unlikely to be very dehydrated, is often sweating profusely, and though the urine may give a positive test with Clinitest,* it will be negative with Clinistix*; similarly, it may give a false positive ferric chloride test for ketones, but will be negative to Ketostix* and Acetest.* Head injury and subarachnoid haemorrhage may be associated with hyperglycaemia and glycosuria, but they are usually easily distinguished by the history, the presence of other neurological signs, and the absence of dehydration and ketonuria.

It is equally important to remember that the diabetic is as prone to these other conditions as anyone else, and not to attribute symptoms to diabetes when they are due to something else. It may be important for example to check for ketonuria in the diabetic with pneumonia, because overbreathing may be thought to be due to diabetic ketosis, when in fact the diabetic upset may be relatively slight, and the overbreathing due to hypoxia. Hypoglycaemic coma is usually easily distinguished from diabetic coma by its rapid onset which may be within minutes of the onset of symptoms, and by remembering that it has none of the characteristic features of diabetic coma. If in doubt a rapid estimation of the blood sugar using Dextrostix* can be helpful.

It is most important to remember the cardinal signs of severe

---

*Ames Company, Stoke Poges, Buckinghamshire, and Elkhart, Indiana.

diabetic keto-acidosis — severe dehydration, rapid breathing and the smell of acetone — which distinguish it from most other causes of coma.

Treatment of Severe Diabetic Keto-acidosis. Having made a diagnosis of diabetic precoma or coma it is prudent to make a personal telephone call to the laboratory staff to inform them of the situation, and to let them know the biochemical estimations that are likely to be required over the next few hours. Co-operation between the biochemist and the clinician is absolutely essential, and if a technician is to undertake emergency estimations which will take him away from other work, or require his working during the night, it is only fair to warn him in advance. He is an essential part of the team.

Before starting treatment arterial blood should be taken for estimation of pH, PCO_2 and PO_2, and this sample may also be used for blood glucose, sodium, potassium, bicarbonate urea, and any other relevant estimations (e.g. serum transaminases, lactic acid, blood culture). Urine should be obtained, preferably without catheterization, as soon as possible, and tested for glucose and ketones, and this should be repeated 4-hourly. *If ketonuria is only slight, but acidosis is evident, lactic acidosis may be present.*

Insulin. Soluble insulin is the only insulin to use in emergencies, because of its rapid action. It is usually best to wait until the blood sugar is known before giving any insulin, though, where delay in obtaining the blood sugar is anticipated, and the clinical diagnosis is undoubted, it is safe to give 30 units of soluble insulin intravenously, and 30 units intramuscularly to an adult, having taken blood for the laboratory. When the blood sugar is known the insulin dose can be based upon it, using the 'Ten per cent rule'. Thus, the dose of insulin, in units, is equal to 10% of the blood sugar level in mg per 100 ml. For example, if the blood sugar is 800 mg per 100 ml, 80 units of soluble insulin are given. One half is given intravenously, because of poor peripheral circulation, and the rest intramuscularly or subcutaneously. (If the entire dose is given intravenously its rapid degradation by the liver, and excretion by the kidneys necessitates giving the next dose not more than 2 hours later.) Subsequent doses can usually be given entirely intramuscularly or subcutaneously. This dose regime is much lower than is used in some centres, particularly in the United States. However, the blood sugar usually falls by about 50% within 4 hours when insulin is given by the '10% rule', which is a perfectly adequate rate of fall. Indeed, there is a distinct danger that a more abrupt fall of plasma glucose and osmolality may result in a shift of water into brain cells, resulting in cerebral oedema (see p. 160). In addition there is a greater chance of hypoglycaemia developing later, when insulin antagonism is overcome, if very large or frequent doses of insulin have been given.

The blood sugar should be re-estimated 2 hours after the first dose of insulin, to make sure that an adequate response has been obtained. If the blood sugar has fallen by 25% or more within 2 hours, no insulin need be given at this time; the next dose is given 4 hours after the first, and is calculated by the 10% rule, from the blood sugar at this time. Thereafter insulin is given 4 hourly.

Example:

Time	0	2 hrs	4 hrs	8 hrs
Blood sugar (mg per 100 ml)	820	605	400	180
Insulin (units)	82	—	40	According to sliding scale.

If, on the other hand, the 2 hour blood sugar has dropped by *less* than 25% of the initial value, the next dose of insulin should be given then, and the blood sugar repeated 2 hours later. Thereafter insulin can usually be given 4 hourly.

Example:

Time	0	2 hrs	4 hrs	6 hrs	10 hrs
Blood sugar (mg per 100 ml)	860	800	580	420	230
Insulin (units)	86	80	—	42	According to sliding scale

In very rare cases in which the blood sugar fails to drop by 25% even after 2 doses of insulin given 2 hours apart, 2-hourly insulin must be continued, but in doses greater than indicated by the 10% rule, until a drop of 25% or more or the initial value has occurred; thereafter it can be given 4-hourly according to the 10% rule.

When the blood sugar has fallen to 300 mg per 100 ml or less, the 4-hourly insulin can be given according to a sliding scale based on the amount of glycosuria. A suitable regime in most cases would be:

Urine glucose	*Insulin dosage* (units)
1–2% with ketonuria	28–36
1–2% without ketonuria	20–28
½–¾%	12–20
Trace–¼%	8–12
Nil	0–8

Twice or thrice daily soluble insulin should be resumed as soon as intravenous fluids are discontinued and the patient is taking his usual carbohydrate allowance by mouth.

Fluids. Usually 6–7 litres of fluid will be required during the first 24 hours in patients with diabetic coma or precoma. Normal saline is *not* the best fluid to use, since losses of sodium exceed those of chloride, and since water losses are relatively greater than electrolyte losses. Saline-lactate solutions have been used, but the use of lactate has certain disadvantages. Lactate is metabolized to bicarbonate, and at a low blood pH this conversion may be impaired. Furthermore high levels of lactate have been demonstrated in some cases of diabetic coma. Glucose-containing fluids should clearly not be used in the initial stages, as they obscure the effects of insulin, may add to the osmotic diuresis, and accelerate the fall of serum potassium. Fructose is of no value in diabetic ketosis, as under these conditions it is largely converted to glucose.

A slightly hypotonic solution, containing more sodium than chloride is required, and a useful solution is shown in Table II.

This solution is available commercially (Boots Co. Nottingham) or can be made up in hospital pharmacies. Hartmann's solution is a suitable substitute, being of the following composition:

TABLE II. Diabetic coma solution

	Na (mEq)	Cl (mEq)	Bicarb (mEq)
660 ml N.saline	102	102	
200 ml 1·3% Na.bicarb	30	—	30
140 ml water	—	—	—
100 ml	132	102	30

(Na, 131 mEq/l; K, 5 mEq/l; Ca, 4 mEq/l; Cl, 111 mEq/l; Bicarb, 29 mEq/l).

Fluid should initially be given rapidly — at a rate of about 1 litre in 30 minutes in an adult unless there are contraindications such as old age or heart disease. This rapid rate of infusion is continued *until clinical signs of dehydration begin to lessen.* Since patients are often hypothermic it is reasonable to warm the fluid to body temperature when it is being given rapidly. It is important to keep the patient warm. All too often, because of frequent examinations and other procedures patients are left exposed unnecessarily. In cases of extreme acidosis, where the serum bicarbonate initially is less than 5 mEq per litre, or the arterial pH less than 7·0, or if, after 2 or 3 hours' treatment a rapid respiration rate due to acidosis has not begun to slow, an additional 100 mEq of sodium bicarbonate may be given (100 ml of 8·4% sodium bicarbonate). It may however be unwise to attempt further correction of acidosis with bicarbonate at this stage. This is because rapid correction of metabolic acidosis with bicarbonate may result in a rise in blood pH while the CSF pH actually *falls* further. This situation seems to arise from an increase in blood pCO_2 as hyperventilation is reduced. This causes a rapid rise in CSF pCO_2, but changes in blood bicarbonate do not affect the CSF bicarbonate so quickly. Hence CSF pCO_2 may rise without significant change in CSF bicarbonate, and CSF acidosis increases. The CSF pH seems to correlate closely with the mental state, so that delayed return to consciousness may be anticipated if too much bicarbonate is given too quickly.

In very rare cases in which severe hypotension persists after 3–4 hours of treatment, whole blood or dextran may be

required to expand the blood volume. Under these circumstances the central venous pressure should be monitored to
avoid overloading the system.

When the blood sugar has fallen to 300 mg per 100 ml or
less, 5% dextrose in water, or 4·3% dextrose in 1/5 normal
saline should be given. As by this time rehydration is usually
nearly complete it may be given at a rate of about 1 litre per
8 hours, which supplies 150 g of glucose per day. Oral fluids
can usually be started within 24 hours, and the normal diet
resumed within 2 or 3 days.

Cutting down on veins to insert a cannula should be avoided
whenever possible in diabetics, as it is important not to destroy
their veins, which may be needed again.

Potassium. The serum potassium is usually normal, or high on
admission, largely as a result of dehydration; sodium depletion,
increased protein breakdown, and diminished glycogen synthesis also tend to raise the serum potassium. The total body
potassium however, is low, so potassium replacement is needed,
usually after about 3 hours of fluid replacement, to prevent
hypokalaemia. Replacement of potassium should not usually
exceed a rate of 25 mEq per hour (2 g KCl per hour), except in
very rare cases where the serum potassium is actually low on
admission in spite of dehydration, signifying a very gross potassium deficit. Under these circumstances potassium replacement
should be started at once, giving 50 mEq (4 g KCl) hourly for
the first 2 hours. The serum potassium should then be measured
2 hours after the start of treatment, and 4 hours thereafter. The
usual case requires about 150—200 mEq of potassium (12—16 g
KCl) in the first 24 hours. ECG tracings may also be used to
detect hypokalaemia (depressed ST segments, inverted T waves,
prolonged PR and QT interval with U waves), and the deep
tendon reflexes may also give a clue to the development of
severe hypokalaemia. This should be suspected if the reflexes,
initially present, are lost in spite of a return to consciousness.
Particular care must be taken in giving potassium to the
occasional patient whose urinary output is poor; otherwise
hyperkalaemia may develop. Fortunately, however, oliguric
renal failure is very rarely seen in diabetic coma, in spite of the
hypotension, probably being prevented by the osmotic diuresis

produced by the hyperglycaemia. Nevertheless, if it does occur haemodialysis may be required.

Emptying the Stomach. The stomach should be aspirated in all unconscious patients, and in those with a succussion splash due to a dilated stomach, in order to reduce the risk of inhalation of vomit. It is not necessary (and it is very unpleasant for the patient) to pass a stomach-tube into someone who is conscious, with severe dehydration and hyperventilation, unless the stomach is dilated.

Treatment of Infection. Any obvious infection, which may have precipitated ketoacidosis, should be treated preferably with a broad-spectrum bactericidal antibiotic given intravenously, until the sensitivity of the organism is known. It is wise to take a blood culture first. The use of antibiotics prophylactically in all unconscious patients has not been shown to be beneficial.

Catheterization. Urethral catheterization should be avoided if possible, and not done merely in order to obtain urine for testing. A blood sugar is more accurate and does not expose the patient to the risk of urinary infection.

Oxygen. The arterial pO_2 is not infrequently lowered in diabetic coma; this may diminish oxygen transport to the tissues, which may already be oxygen deficient due to the reduced blood volume. Administration of oxygen seems to be well justified in the early stages of treatment, unless the pO_2 is known to be over 80 mm Hg.

Summary of Treatment
1. Take a brief history and examine the patient. Note the level of consciousness, state of hydration, and the smell of acetone. Record temperature, pulse rate, respiration rate and blood pressure. Check the tendon reflexes, test for a succussion splash, and look for infection.
2. Take arterial blood for pH, pCO_2, O_2, glucose, sodium, potassium, bicarbonate, urea, and any other relevant estimations.

157

3. Test urine for sugar and ketones and repeat 4-hourly, avoiding catheterization if possible.

4. *Insulin.* Give that number of units of soluble insulin which is equal to 10% of the blood sugar in mg per 100 ml (half intravenously; half intramuscularly).

   Measure blood sugar 2 hours after first dose of insulin. *If it has fallen by 25%* or more, give no insulin then. Repeat blood sugar 4 hours after start of treatment, and give insulin then and 4-hourly, according to 10% rule.

   If blood sugar has fallen by less than 25% at 2 hours, give insulin then, according to 10% rule based on second blood sugar. Thereafter give insulin 4-hourly according to blood sugar, until this is down to 300 mg per 100 ml.

   When blood sugar falls below 300 mg per 100 ml give insulin 4-hourly according to sliding scale based on quantity of urinary glucose (see p. 154).

5. *Fluids.*
   (a) *Saline-bicarbonate.* Start with infusion of diabetic coma, solution (see p. 155), and run at 1 litre per 30 minutes in adults, until dehydration lessens (unless patient is aged or has heart disease). Warm fluid to body temperature. If initial arterial pH less than 7·1, or if rapid respiration not reduced after 3 hours' treatment, give 100 mEq sodium bicarbonate.

   (b) *Glucose-saline.* When blood sugar down to 300 mg per 100 ml, give 5% dextrose in water or 4·3% dextrose in 1/5 normal saline, and if rehydrated run at 1 litre per 8 hours.

6. *Potassium.* Start replacing potassium after 2 hours treatment; (if serum potassium subnormal start immediately). Do not exceed a rate of 25 mEq per hour (2 g KCl per hour) unless initial serum potassium subnormal — if so, give at rate of 4 g KCl per hour for 2 hours. Measure serum potassium 2 hours after start of treatment and 4 hours later. About 12–16 g KCl usually required in first 24 hours.

7. *Aspirate the stomach* in unconscious patients, and those with succussion splash.

8. *Antibiotics*. Treat overt infection with broad-spectrum bactericidal antibiotic until sensitivities known.
9. Give oxygen by mask until patient is conscious, and keep patient warm.

Prevention of Diabetic Ketosis

The majority of diabetics admitted to hospital in severe keto-acidosis have either failed to increase their insulin to meet an increased demand caused by intercurrent illness, or have actually omitted their insulin. Diabetic coma arising under these circumstances is preventable if patients are properly taught how to manage their diabetes. Only too commonly a patient will explain that he stopped his insulin because he was not eating normally, or because he was vomiting, and thought that his insulin would not therefore be required. Occasionally patients have even been advised to stop their insulin under these circumstances by a doctor. Such a course of action in the insulin-dependent diabetic will inevitably lead to diabetic ketosis.

Patients should be advised that if they are not eating properly because of some intercurrent infection, they should take their usual carbohydrate allowance as fluids, which can often be tolerated when solids cannot. One tablespoonful of Ribena, 4 tablespoonsful of Lucozade, or 2 teaspoonsful of sugar dissolved in water flavoured with diabetic squash, will each provide approximately 10 g of carbohydrate, and can be used in place of solids.

The urine must be tested twice daily, and the insulin dose must be increased if 1−2% glycosuria develops in the presence of infection. For most adults on twice daily soluble insuline, an increase of about 8 units on each successive dose until there is less than 1% glycosuria, usually brings the situation under control. If it does not do so rapidly an extra dose of about 8 units of soluble insulin should be given before the midday meal as long as there is 1−2% glycosuria at that time. For diabetics on a single injection of soluble plus a long-acting insulin, whose urine tests both before breakfast and the evening meal show 1−2% glucose, the soluble insulin should be increased by about 8 units in the morning, and an additional 8 units should be given before the evening meal. Daily increments in the dose may be required

159

until there is less than 1% glycosuria. Increasing the dose of a daily injection of Lente or Isophane insulin is often not very effective in overcoming a rapid increase in insulin requirement, and if control is not quickly achieved by so doing, it is wise to switch temporarily to twice daily soluble insulin. If, in spite of these measures diabetes remains uncontrolled, and particularly if there is continued vomiting, the patient should be in hospital.

About a quarter of the patients admitted to hospital in diabetic coma or pre-coma are new diabetics, previously un-diagnosed. Symptoms of diabetes have usually been present for several days, or weeks, before consciousness is lost, and as urine is plentiful during this time, and tests for sugar and ketones easy, diagnosis should be possible before the patient is comatose.

Cerebral Oedema in Diabetic Coma

Cerebral oedema is a very unusual but highly dangerous compli-cation of diabetic coma, which has been reported with increasing frequency over the last ten years. It is a particularly tragic situa-tion as it is almost always fatal, usually occurs in adolescents or young adults, and should be preventable. It has usually been described in patients who initially respond well to treatment. The usual biochemical measurements are returning towards normal, and the state of consciousness improving when the patient rather abruptly loses consciousness again and dies with cerebral oedema. There seem to be no clinical features at the outset which differentiate these patients from those who recover.

It is known that cerebral blood flow falls in acidosis, and that cerebral utilization of oxygen is reduced. This results in cerebral hypoxia. Acute hypoxia is associated with an increase in cerebral venous potassium and a decrease in cerebral venous sodium without significant change in cerebral arterial electro-lytes. This suggests that the brain gains sodium and loses potas-sium in these conditions.

Cerebral oedema has however been reported in patients dying in aketotic coma, so some mechanism other than acidosis must sometimes be involved. Hyperglycaemia increases the synthesis of sorbitol and fructose in brain cells in animals, and since sorbitol and fructose cross cell membranes slowly, it is likely that if the blood glucose is *rapidly* lowered, intracellular hyperosmolarity would occur, producing a sudden shift of water into brain cells. Indeed rapid falls of blood glucose are now known to be associated with the development of abnormally high CSF pressure. This underlines the importance of reducing blood glucose relatively slowly as is usually ensured using a 10% rule for insulin dosage.

If the development of cerebral oedema can be recognized in time the prompt use of intravenous mannitol is recommended, to extract fluid from the cells.

DIABETIC COMA WITHOUT KETO-ACIDOSIS (HYPEROSMOLAR, NON-KETOTIC COMA)

Diabetic coma may occur in the absence of keto-acidosis, and this is sometimes referred to as hyperosmolar coma. The condition usually occurs in patients over 50, in contrast to ketotic coma which is more commonly seen in younger patients. It has however been reported in children. Patients developing aketotic coma are usually not previously known to be diabetic, which may account for delay in making the diagnosis. This, together with the older age of these patients probably accounts for its high mortality, which may be up to 50%. A curious thing about aketotic coma is that not infrequently patients do not require insulin subsequently, indicating that endogenous insulin is available, in contrast to the situation in keto-acidotic coma.

The clinical picture of aketotic coma includes very severe dehydration, and because there is no acidosis there is neither hyperventilation nor a smell of acetone on the breath. The diagnosis is therefore more difficult than in the ketotic patient, and more easily confused with a cerebro-vascular catastrophe, particularly as convulsions may occur in these patients. Dehydration is the clue, and *the unconscious, elderly patient who is profoundly dehydrated needs a blood glucose estimation.*

The most striking biochemical abnormality is the extremely high blood sugar, which may be related to the huge quantities of sugary drinks these patients have often been taking. In many cases the blood sugar is over 1000 mg per 100 ml, whereas levels this high are uncommon in patients with ketotic coma. Serum osmolality is therefore also very high in most cases. The blood bicarbonate and pH, however, are within the normal range.

161

Blood insulin levels, while low in relation to the blood sugar level may sometimes be higher than in cases of ketotic coma, and it has been suggested that hyperglycaemia without ketosis may be due to dissociation of the effects of *small* quantities of insulin on glucose uptake on the one hand, and fatty acid release on the other. Thus there may be sufficient insulin to inhibit lipolysis, yet not enough for normal glucose utilization. In many cases, however, the serum insulin is similar to that in ketotic coma. The known antiketogenic effect of extreme hyper-glycaemia may also be implicated in some cases, but cannot be the only explanation for the condition, as the blood sugar is not always remarkably high. Alternatively, lack of ketosis might be due to a block in the pathway leading to ketogenesis in the liver.

Treatment. A large volume of hypotonic saline, such as ½-normal saline, is required to combat the hyperosmolality. Normal saline is likely to precipitate severe hypernatraemia. Large doses of insulin may be hazardous in aketotic coma, because of the lack of the insulin antagonism associated with ketosis; but insulin given according to the 10% rule appears to be safe. There is justification for the use of anticoagulants in hyperosmolar patients, who are at considerable risk of thrombotic episodes.

LACTIC ACIDOSIS

Lactic acidosis is uncommon, but when it occurs it is often in association with diabetic ketosis complicated by severe tissue hypoxia resulting from circulatory failure. It may therefore be seen in association with shock, for example from myocardial infarction, pulmonary embolism, haemorrhage or septicaemia, or in patients with renal failure. Where the arterial pH is unexpectedly low for the degree of ketonaemia or where the 'anion gap' ([sodium plus potassium] minus [chloride plus bicarbonate]), in mEq per litre is more than 20, lactic acidosis should be suspected. Clinically these patients resemble diabetics with keto-acidosis. Treatment includes correction of the acidosis with sodium bicarbonate. The bicarbonate requirement can be calculated from the equation of Mellengaard and Astrup:

mEq HCO_3 required = 0·3 X Body wt. (kg) X Base deficit (mEq per litre).

Usually only about 1/3 of this calculated requirement should be replaced initially. Efforts must also be made to maintain tissue perfusion, care being taken not to overload the patient, which requires monitoring the central venous pressure. Oxygen should also be given. The prognosis is very poor and as these patients are often resistant to treatment with bicarbonate, haemodialysis should be considered early.

HYPOGLYCAEMIA

Loss of consciousness in a diabetic on insulin must always suggest hypoglycaemia. This is usually, but not always, preceded by symptoms including anxiety and confusion, irritability or frank aggression, shakiness, sweating and hunger. Less common manifestations of hypoglycaemia include paraesthesiae around the mouth, transient diplopia or dysarthria, and sudden hemiplegia, usually rapidly reversible. Such reactions to insulin are most likely to occur before lunch or around bedtime in patients on twice daily soluble insulin, but arise at more variable times in patients on long-acting insulins, occurring usually in the afternoon, evening or night. Headache, sometimes accompanied by nausea, occurring in the early mornings in patients on a long-acting insulin should suggest nocturnal hypoglycaemia.

Symptoms due to hypoglycaemia may be due to other causes than exogenous insulin. Occasionally oral sulphonylureas, particularly chlorpropamide given to elderly malnourished patients, may produce severe hypoglycaemia. Sulphonylurea induced hypoglycaemia is particularly dangerous because it may be protracted, and may recur over a few days unless steps are taken to prevent this. Hypoglycaemia has also been present intermittently for many years in a large proportion of patients ultimately found to have insulinomas. Frequently in these patients classical hypoglycaemic symptoms are denied, and hypoglycaemia shows itself only in periodic, and variable disturbances of behaviour ranging from restlessness and aggression to more bizarre forms of inappropriate behaviour. The fact that neuro-psychiatric symptoms may persist beyond the period of hypoglycaemia, has

163

resulted in the diagnosis being missed and some of these unfortunate people have been treated for years as psychotics.

Reactive hypoglycaemia usually occurs 2—3 hours after meals, in contrast to the fasting hypoglycaemia commonly seen in patients with insulinomas. Hypoglycaemic symptoms usually 3—4 hours after meals may also precede the development of diabetes, and hypoglycaemia may also occur in hypopituitarism, hypoadrenalism, and very occasionally in patients with severe liver disease, large, usually retroperitoneal fibromas or sarcomas, or after an alcoholic bout in the malnourished.

Treatment. Emergency treatment of hypoglycaemia is simple and rewarding. Usually 20 g of glucose, given intravenously if the patient is not sufficiently conscious to take it by mouth, is adequate, but severe insulin reactions may, occasionally, require much more — even up to 100 g of glucose. Diabetics suffering from sulphonylurea-induced hypoglycaemia should continue to take 20 g of carbohydrate 2-hourly after regaining consciousness, including during the night, until there is persistent glycosuria, because of the risk of recurrent hypoglycaemia. Occasionally glucagon can be invaluable for the treatment of hypoglycaemia. Glucagon raises the blood sugar by releasing glucose from liver glycogen, and in a small child, convulsing from hypoglycaemia, where oral glucose is impossible to give, and intravenous glucose difficult, 1·0 mg of glucagon intramuscularly or subcutaneously will usually raise the blood sugar sufficiently to restore consciousness. Oral glucose should be given as soon as possible thereafter, as the effect of glucagon is transient, and relapse into unconsciousness will otherwise occur.

Prevention. At attempt should always be made to ascertain the cause of hypoglycaemia, in order to prevent its recurrence. Most commonly in insulin-dependent diabetics it is delay in a mealtime, or unusual exertion which precipitates hypoglycaemia, but there are other less common causes. For example, insulin is poorly absorbed if given habitually into the same site, particularly if given into areas of insulin hypertrophy, and a change from such a site to a normal area may result in hypoglycaemia. The insulin strength should be checked to make sure the patient on 40 units per ml insulin has not inadvertently been given 80 units per ml strength. The injection technique should be observed, to ensure that the plunger of the syringe is being withdrawn to avoid injecting intravenously. If no cause is evident, and particularly if hypoglycaemic episodes have been occurring frequently, the dose of insulin must be reduced.

THYROID CRISIS

Thyroid crisis, or storm, is a life-threatening and sudden exacerbation of all the symptoms and signs of thyrotoxicosis. It cannot be ascribed merely to an abrupt increase in the release of thyroid hormones, though, since poorly controlled thyrotoxics exposed to thyroidectomy are particularly at risk of thyroid crisis, this may be one factor contributing to the condition. Nowadays, as patients are usually euthyroid before thyroidectomy, thyroid crisis is seen more frequently when poorly controlled or untreated thyrotoxics are exposed to other stresses, such as any major surgery, trauma, severe infections, myocardial infarction, or even serious emotional upsets. Under these circumstances there is enhanced activity of the sympathetic nervous system and increased release of catecholamines into the circulation. In the thyrotoxic there is an increase in circulating free catecholamines and thyroid crisis may be partly due to this.

Clinical Picture. The patient is apprehensive, restless, irritable and breathing rapidly. A high temperature is characteristic, and because sweating is often profuse at first, the patient becomes dehydrated. The pulse rate may rise to 150—200 per minute, and rapid atrial fibrillation is common. Heart failure may develop. Diarrhoea and mild jaundice are sometimes seen. The patient ultimately becomes shocked and comatose.

Laboratory tests of thyroid function will confirm the diagnosis, and blood should be taken for these measurements, but treatment must not wait upon the results when a clinical diagnosis of thyroid crisis has been made.

Treatment. Reduction in sympathetic overactivity may be achieved with propranolol, which blocks β-adrenergic receptors,

165

with intramuscular reserpine, which depletes tissue catecholamines, or with guanethidine, which both depletes catecholamine
stores, and blocks sympathetic transmission. None of these agents
affects thyroid function, but all are effective in treating thyroid
crisis, and one should be chosen. Administration is as follows:

Propranolol. 1—2 mg *slowly* intravenously, followed by 40 mg
8-hourly, orally or via a naso-gastric tube. NB. This may exacer-
bate or precipitate cardiac failure, and digitalis may be required
in addition.

Reserpine. 1—5 mg intramuscularly, repeated 4—6-hourly.
NB. This should be avoided if the patient is hypotensive.

Guanethidine. 25—50 mg 6-hourly orally, or via a naso-gastric
tube. NB. This should be avoided if the patient is hypotensive.

Measures to reduce thyroid hormone release must also be
taken. Sodium iodide, placed in the intravenous fluid, and given
at a rate of 1—2 g 6-hourly will promptly inhibit thyroid
hormone secretion, and subsequently can be replaced by Lugols
iodine by mouth (10 drops 8-hourly). As soon as possible
carbimazole, 15 mg 8-hourly orally, should be started, though
its effects on thyroid hormone secretion are delayed.

As the patient is usually dehydrated 4·3% glucose in 1/5
normal saline is required intravenously, but because of the risk
of cardiac failure, central venous pressure monitoring may be
needed. Excessively rapid catabolism of cortisol may lead to a
relative deficiency of this hormone, and 100 mg of cortisol 6-
hourly should be given initially, especially if the patient is
shocked. Water soluble vitamins, especially B vitamins, may be
deficient, and should also be given. The patient should be cooled
by means of fans and cool sponging.

The cause of the crisis must be sought, particular attention
being directed to the prompt treatment of any underlying infection.

With such treatment the crisis should be over in 3 or 4 days,
though occasionally it lasts longer.

ACUTE ADRENAL INSUFFICIENCY

Acute adrenal insufficiency occurs when the adrenal glands fail
to produce sufficient glucocorticoid and mineralocorticoid

hormones in response to stress. This may arise when acute
adrenal haemorrhage, fulminating infection, trauma, or thrombosis, affect previously normal adrenals, or when stressful
situations occur in patients with chronically diseased adrenals,
such as those with Addison's disease, or those whose adrenals
are suppressed by prolonged corticosteroid therapy. In the latter
the maintenance dosage of adrenal corticosteroids may be
adequate under normal circumstances, but inadequate to cope
with sudden superimposed stress, such as surgery, infection or
trauma.

Clinical Picture

The patient with acute adrenal insufficiency is gravely ill, with
nausea, vomiting, profound weakness, and hypotension due to a
shift of sodium and water from the intravascular to the intracellular space, as well as to loss of sodium in the urine due to
lack of aldosterone. In Addison's disease, pigmentation of the
skin and mucous membranes may be evident. In children and
young adults meningococcaemia may be associated with adrenal
haemorrhage, and generalized purpura and fever are characteristic
additional signs.

Blood should be taken for estimation of the serum electrolytes, blood count, blood urea and glucose, and plasma cortisol.
Hyponatraemia and hyperkalaemia are characteristic, though
occasionally the serum sodium is normal because of haemo-
concentration. The total eosinophil count is high — it may be
above 50 per mm^3 — though a lower level does not exclude
adrenal insufficiency. Hypoglycaemia and moderate azotaemia
may occur, and plasma cortisol is low, or low relative to the
stress.

Treatment. Acute adrenal insufficiency demands provision of
adequate amounts of cortisol and mineralocorticoid, and
sufficient sodium and water to combat shock and dehydration.
Hypoglycaemia must be corrected, and infection treated. The
pulse and blood pressure must be recorded hourly or half-
hourly, and central venous pressure monitoring is helpful to
prevent fluid overload.

Hydrocortisone hemisuccinate is given immediately in a dose

of 100 mg intravenously, and 50 mg are given 6-hourly there-after in the intravenous infusion for the first 24 hours. The intravenous infusion of 5% dextrose in *normal* saline should be run rapidly at first, the first litre being given in about one hour. Three or four litres are likely to be required in the first 24 hours. Mineralocorticoid, such as desoxycorticosterone acetate or 9-α fluorohydrocortisone are not required at first, because sufficiently large doses of cortisol are being given to provide adequate mineralocorticoid action.

On the second day cortisone acetate can usually be given by mouth in a dose of 50 mg 6-hourly, and the intravenous fluid can usually be reduced to about half that required in the first 24 hours. Thereafter intravenous fluids can usually be dis-continued, and the dose of cortisone acetate gradually reduced over 4 or 5 days to a maintenance dose of 12·5 mg 8-hourly. For adequate sodium retention 9-α fluorohydrocortisone, in a dose of 0·1 mg daily by mouth is added when the cortisone acetate has been reduced to about 75 mg per day.

Hypotension in hypoadrenalism responds poorly to vaso-pressors which are best avoided. If shock is unusually prolonged larger doses of hydrocortisone may be required, and plasma or dextran may very occasionally be needed to expand the blood volume.

It must be emphasized to the patient that the dose of corti-sone should be doubled or trebled in times of stress such as with infections or surgery. A 'steroid card' indicating details of treatment should be provided.

SECONDARY HYPOADRENALISM

A similar clinical state may arise in the patient with adrenal insufficiency secondary to pituitary disease, though it is usually less severe than primary hypoadrenalism, as adrenal aldosterone production is little affected, at least in the early stages of pituitary insufficiency. Hypoglycaemia however may be severe, as insulin sensitivity is increased by lack of growth hormone as well as lack of cortisol.

The patient usually has signs of long-standing deficiencies of pituitary hormones. Thus there is usually pallor out of propor-tion to the anaemia, and the areolae of the breasts are pale (lack of ACTH and MSH); there is lack of pubic and axillary hair and atrophy of the external genitalia (lack of gonadotropins); there may be signs of hypothyroidism (lack of thyrotropin), though swelling of the subcutaneous tissue is usually less obvious than in primary hypothyroidism. Lack of growth hormone and gonadotropins may both contribute to the fineness and excessive wrinkling of the skin, particularly noticeable around the mouth.

Treatment. Treatment of acute secondary adrenal insufficiency is as for primary adrenal insufficiency, but replacement of thyroid hormone, and sometimes gonadal hormones, will be required later.

MYXOEDEMA COMA

This is a rare condition, usually seen in elderly women, which must be considered in the differential diagnosis of coma, especially when there is hypothermia. Stupor or coma is commonly precipitated by some stressful situation, not uncommonly exposure to cold, or by sedative or narcotic drugs to which these patients are unusually sensitive. Signs of long-standing, severe hypothyroidism are evident, and particularly helpful clues are hypothermia without shivering, bradycardia, bradypnoea, and constipation.

Laboratory tests confirm hypothyroidism, and usually reveal anaemia; in some cases hyponatraemia, hypochloraemia, respiratory acidosis and hypoglycaemia are seen. The cerebrospinal fluid protein may be raised; the ECG reveals bradycardia and low voltage, and the chest X-ray may show a pericardial effusion.

Treatment. The mortality is around 70%, and a most important factor in survival is the *prompt* institution of thyroid hormone in *low* dosage. This means that rapidly acting triiodothyronine is preferred to thyroxine. It is however unwise to give triiodothyronine intravenously, or in high dosage, because of the risk of inducing cardiac dysrhythmias, such as atrial fibrillation or ventricular tachycardia, or angina and cardiac failure. Absorption of triiodothyronine from the gastro-intestinal tract is prompt, and recovery is usually rapid in cases treated with triiodothyronine via a naso-gastric tube, so that there seems to be no need to give it intravenously. It is recommended that 10 μg dissolved in saline be given 12-hourly via a naso-gastric tube at first. The dose should be increased *gradually,* depending upon the pulse rate, as many of these patients have associated heart disease. The return to a normal metabolic rate is likely to provoke adrenal insufficiency in a patient with long-standing primary myxoedema, and even more so in one with hypothyroidism secondary to pituitary disease, so adrenal steroids must be given with the triiodothyronine. Hydrocortisone, 100 mg intravenously initially and 50 mg 6-hourly for the next 24 hours is recommended, with a gradual reduction thereafter.

Hypoglycaemia may require intravenous glucose, but care should be taken in giving intravenous saline in primary myxoedema, even when there is hyponatraemia, as the total body sodium tends to be high, and serum sodium rises with thyroid replacement as sodium and water are released from connective tissue. Bradypnoea with resultant respiratory acidosis may necessitate assisted ventilation, and vigorous suction of the bronchial tree to get rid of mucus.

HYPERCALCAEMIC CRISIS

The commonest causes of severe hypercalcaemia are hyperparathyroidism, and osteolytic bone metastases, especially from breast cancer. Hypercalcaemic crisis is associated with a variety of symptoms, including generalized muscular weakness, anorexia, nausea and vomiting, polyuria and polydipsia, dehydration, weight loss and cardiac irregularities. Ultimately lethargy, stupor or coma develop. An increase in bone pain commonly accompanies hypercalcaemia due to bone metastases. Hypercalcaemic crisis is likely to arise when the serum calcium is above 16 mg per 100 ml.

Treatment. Intravenous saline is required for rehydration, and this also encourages a calcium diuresis. At least 3 litres daily is usually required. A low calcium diet and an oral neutral phosphate mixture* (60 ml 8-hourly) help to reduce the serum calcium, but in a serious emergency when the patient cannot be fed orally, an intravenous infusion of phosphate may be required. This facilitates deposition of calcium in bone and other tissues, but should be given with great caution if hypocalcaemia is to be avoided. A suitable regime is to give 500 ml of 0·1 M phosphate buffer, made up of disodium phosphate (0·081 M) and monopotassium phosphate (0·019 M), intravenously over 12 hours. This supplies 1·55 g of phosphorus. Depending upon the response a further 500 ml may be given.

Alternatively, intravenous isotonic sodium sulphate (3·85 per cent) may be used. This increases the urinary loss of calcium, and 2—3 litres may be given in 8—12 hours, taking care to avoid sodium overload and potassium deficit, the latter being due to urinary potassium loss.

Corticosteroids have a delayed hypocalcaemic action, but are rarely effective in hypercalcaemia due either to hyperparathyroidism or bone secondaries.

If the acute crisis is due to hyperparathyroidism, parathyroidectomy is necessary as soon as possible. If it is due to bone secondaries the oral neutral phosphate mixture may be required after the acute crisis is over.

ACUTE HYPOCALCAEMIA

Acute hypocalcaemia with tetany may develop after parathyroidectomy where there is extensive bone disease, as calcium is rapidly taken up by the 'hungry bones' after the parathyroid adenoma is removed. This can usually be remedied with a continuous infusion of calcium gluconate, giving 100 ml 10% calcium gluconate in 900 ml of 5% dextrose in water each day, until the serum calcium remains within the normal range. Occasionally larger amounts of calcium are required. Acute hypocalcaemia due to other causes is also treated with calcium gluconate intravenously, though usually a prolonged infusion is not required,

Neutral Phosphate Mixture.
Na_2HPO_4 (Anhydrous) 3·66 g.
$NaH_2PO_4 . 2H_2O$ 1 g.
Orange syrup 16 ml.
Purified water to 60 ml.

171

and other treatment, including vitamin D may subsequently be needed, depending upon the cause of the hypocalcaemia.

FURTHER READING

Sheldon, J., and Pyke, D. A. (1968). Severe diabetic ketosis: precoma and coma. In *Clinical Diabetes and its Biochemical Basis.* Ed. Oakley, W. G., Pyke, D. A., and Taylor, K. W. Blackwell Scientific Publications.

Hockaday, T. D. R. and Alberti, K. G. M. M. (1972). Diabetic coma, *Brit. J. Hosp. Med.* 7, 183.

Rosenberg, I. N. (1970). Thyroid storm. *New Eng. J. Med.*, 283, 1052.

Hall, R., Anderson, J. and Smart, G. A. (1969). *Fundamentals of Clinical Endocrinology,* Pitman Medical Publishing Co. Ltd.

Perlmutter, M. and Cohn, H. (1964). Myxedema crisis of pituitary or thyroid origin, *Am. J. Med.*, 36, 883.

Thalassinos, N. and Joplin, G. F. (1968). Phosphate treatment of hypercalcaemia due to carcinoma. *Brit. Med. J.*, 4, 14.

Benvenisti, D. S., Sherwood, L. M. and Heinemann, H. O. (1969). Hypercalcaemic crisis in acute leukemia, *Am. J. Med.*, 46, 976.

Chapter 6

Neurosurgical Conditions

B. CRYMBLE

INTRODUCTION

HEAD INJURIES

Pathology

Scalp injuries
Skull fractures
Cerebral trauma

Resuscitation

The airway
Intubation and tracheostomy
Artificial ventilation
Cerebral death
Circulatory state

Assessment of CNS

Charts, observations and recording
Conscious level
Pupil state
Vital functions
External warning signs
Hemiplegia

173

Special Aspects

> *X-ray examination*
> *Decerebrate rigidity*
> *Cerebral oedema*
> *Head injuries in children*
> *Co-existing injuries*
> *Relief of pain*
> *Post-concussion confusion*

CEREBRAL TUMOUR

SUBARACHNOID HAEMORRHAGE

INTRODUCTION

Neurology units in this country are widely spaced, each one covering a large area and population. Few, if any, of them are in possession of so many beds that all neurological emergencies could be accepted for direct admission, even if such an arrangement were desirable. In fact, the patient's condition is frequently such that a long and immediate journey to a neurological centre would not be in his interests; the more so when, in most cases, the urgent treatment required can be just as readily carried out in any general hospital equipped to deal with emergencies. The greatest anxieties seem to be engendered by those cases in which surgical intervention might be necessary, particularly head injuries, and most junior medical staff are often unsure of themselves when called upon to cope, alone, with the primary management of such patients. This is understandable and largely stems from, at the best, only scant experience of emergency neurology as a student as well as an all too common impression that, except for the few, neurological diagnosis is difficult. Behind all this, in the case of head injuries, lies the uneasy feeling that undeserved medico-legal notoriety can be so readily achieved.

For the casualty officer the text-book emphasis on the undoubtedly important, yet somehow very infrequent, extra-dural haemorrhage is soon overshadowed by the far commoner practical problems of who to X-ray, when to X-ray, who to admit and who to send home when beds are scarce. Other

174

questions which are frequently posed can be mentioned. What is the first thing one should do for the unconscious head-injured patient? What is the significance of a fixed dilated pupil or a pulse rate of 50 per minute in a fully conscious patient? Because of these and many other similar problems no apology is made for being dogmatic on topics which are subjects of debate in neurological circles; it is far more important that the doctor involved should have a few well tried rules of procedure to help him in dealing with such emergencies. Junior medical staff must always remember that they can be expected to go only so far in the management of these patients, but that which is easily within their capabilities in the way of assessment, resuscitation and initiating observations can be of vital importance to the outcome. Contrary to popular belief, a wide knowledge of neurology and the pathology of cerebral trauma is not essential.

In this section the term Intensive Care is given a rather wider meaning than usual. Thus, whilst dealing primarily with the management of obviously ill patients, it is extended to include the care and observation of those many patients with seemingly only mild head injuries who are nevertheless still within that period of time in which complications might develop. In addition, two other emergency neurological conditions are discussed within the limits of what can and should be done when they present in a general hospital, namely: subarachnoid haemorrhage and the urgent deteriorating cerebral tumour. When read at leisure much of what is said might seem to be obvious and unnecessarily stressed. This is done deliberately to emphasize what is in practice so often forgotten in the urgency and isolation of the actual encounter. The emphasis is on assessment for the purpose of immediate and efficient non-operative care of the patient, and, except for one contingency in the case of cerebral tumour, no attempt is made to deal with operative surgical procedures. These are fully covered in the several available works on emergency and neurological surgery.

HEAD INJURIES

The Pathology of Head Injuries

It is necessary to review this topic only in sufficient detail to make the management of head injuries a rational undertaking.

The various forms of primary trauma to the whole head occur at the moment of impact; the scalp is lacerated, the skull is fractured and the brain is damaged — Primary Cerebral Trauma. The effects of any primary cerebral trauma can soon be augmented by complicating processes set in motion by the original injury — Secondary Cerebral Trauma. Thus, damaged cerebral tissue becomes swollen from several causes and torn intracranial blood vessels result in an accumulating haemorrhage. The combined effect of these two processes is a raising of intracranial pressure which, if unrelieved, is soon followed by cerebral displacements.

> *These complications, if they are to develop, almost always show themselves within the first eight hours following injury.*
> *This is the critical period for regular, frequent and accurate observation of the patient.*

Scalp Injuries. Lacerations of the scalp can be very extensive and may result in a heavy and rapid loss of blood, 500—1000 ml being not uncommon. The generous blood supply to the scalp, which results in such substantial haemorrhage, is the reason why there is rarely any tissue loss through ischaemia even when a large scalp flap remains attached by only a relatively small pedicle. Before suturing any scalp lacerations it is important to inspect the base of the wound for bone fragments, a depressed fracture or the escape of CSF or brain tissue.

Skull Fractures. In the vault of the skull fractures may be linear or depressed. Most linear fractures are simple and of very little significance but a few of those occurring in the temporal region cause tearing of an entrapped middle meningeal artery and an extra-dural haemorrhage then rapidly develops. When this occurs blood usually extrudes through the fracture line to accumulate extra-cranially as well as extra-durally; the finding of a boggy swelling in the temporal region is a sign of great importance. On occasions a fracture crossing the vertex can, by tearing adherent dura, result in considerable extra-dural venous haemorrhage from the superior sagittal sinus. Depressed fractures require detection but no further action outside of a neurosurgical unit.

Basal fractures are potentially more serious and are not

uncommonly complicated by tearing of the lining dura mater and its contained venous sinuses, the creation of CSF fistulae and injury to one or more cranial nerves. Coincidental lacerations of the undersurface of the brain are common, and ensuing haemorrhage from torn cerebral vessels and venous sinuses can be profuse. Patients who were wearing crash helmets at the time of their accident can sometimes have surprisingly severe basal and cerebral injuries and yet have neither fractures of the skull vault nor scalp injuries.

Cerebral Injuries. There is a wide range of possible traumatic lesions within the cerebral substance, but there is not always a close correlation between the severity of the injuring forces and the seriousness of the resulting brain damage. The least severe outcome, that of so-called mild concussion, is both the commonest and yet the least understood. It is a clinical phenomenon characterized by a short term of unconsciousness followed by a seemingly full recovery of cerebral functions. The probability is that the essential disturbances in concussion are widespread and intracellular, occurring at a molecular or metabolic level. Many believe that it is the involvement in this disturbance of the cells of the brain stem reticular formations which is responsible for the loss of consciousness. Although the patient's recovery is apparently complete it is more than likely that many neurones fail to survive the injury. Certainly those who have been subjected to repeated concussion have eventually shown unmistakeable signs of cerebral neurone deficiency. The term concussion is generally acknowledged to be imprecise and unsatisfactory, but it must continue to serve until a better understanding of this state has been achieved.

With the impact of the injuring forces on the head the semi-solid brain undergoes a combination of displacement and distortion, and this results in several additional possible types of injury. Distortion of the brain creates shearing stresses which tear both capillaries and neuronal processes, particularly at the grey matter-white matter interface. The capillary disruption produces not only petaechial haemorrhages but also considerable microscopic focal ischaemia, thus adding to the direct neuronal damage. The total volume of these pinpoint multiple haemorrhages can be appreciable, and, in addition, each focus

177

soon becomes surrounded by oedema. As a result brain volume and tension increase which in turn lead to further embarrassment of the cerebral circulation, particularly the venous drainage, and consequently a worsening of any neuro-logical deficits. Sometimes these shearing forces are quite considerable and can result in the tearing of a macroscopic intra-cerebral blood vessel as a result of which a large focal haematoma develops. En masse movement of the brain within the cranial cavity results in cortical contusions, the tearing of cerebral bridging veins and lacerations of the undersurface of the brain as it impacts itself onto the sharp basal ridges of bone and the edges of the dural folds which sub-divide the cranial cavity.

These lesions of the brain and their ensuing effects can set in motion several vicious cycles of events as shown in Fig. 6.1. Treatment is aimed at breaking these cycles and thereby preventing a steady worsening of the brain's condition. Unfortunately, in an appreciable number of cases, the primary injuries are so severe that all attempts at treatment are unavailing.

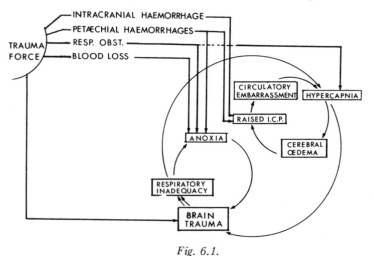

Fig. 6.1.

As a link between this brief survey of the pathology of head injuries and the next section which deals with the practical problems of management it is instructive to review a reasonably large number of cases and see in retrospect just what happened to them. The pattern which emerges is naturally not exactly the same as that which would be found in all parts of the country, but the over-all picture is probably fairly representative. The cases of 500 consecutive head injured patients presenting at hospitals in this area were studied and each patient was placed into one of four groups:

Group A — minor to moderate concussion, admitted for simple treatment and observation only.

Group B — severe concussion or other cerebral injuries but requiring no operative intervention; survived.

Group C — intracranial haemorrhage; were operated upon and recovered.

Group D — severe cerebral injuries and died, with or without operation.

Group	Adults	Children	Total	Approx %	Attention to Airway	Intubation Performed
A	157	221	378	75	40	0
B	67	6	73	15	65	43
C	4	2	6	1	6	6
D	40	3	43	9	43	38

The points to be noted are that 90 per cent of patients survived without the need for any form of neurosurgery but almost one quarter of them required attention to their airways. In contrast, only 1 per cent had cerebral injuries that were benefited by an operation.

MANAGEMENT OF HEAD INJURIES

The management of any condition consists firstly of assessment followed by treatment. When dealing with major forms of trauma the first object of assessment is to determine what steps are necessary for the resuscitation of the patient with particular attention being paid to his respiratory function and circulatory state. This is particularly true of trauma to the central nervous system which is very dependent on these two vital functions for its own activities to continue normally; even an uninjured brain

179

cannot tolerate for very long the biochemical changes brought about by respiratory embarrassment and insufficiency. The effects of primary brain trauma can be considerably aggravated by hypoxia and hypercapnia and no reliable picture of the true extent of brain damage can be obtained until these two factors have been removed. The improvement in CNS function brought about thereby can often be impressive, both in its rapidity and degree. In all cases of head injury therefore the first step should be:

To clear and maintain the airway, assisting respiration if necessary.

The unconscious patient is at great risk of respiratory obstruction, particularly if lying supine. It has been said, and not without some truth, that the patient left in this position, looking up to heaven, will be amongst the first to get there. There is a danger of the tongue falling back and blocking the pharynx, especially in certain forms of mandibular fracture which result in the loss of tongue anchorage in the floor of the mouth. Oro-pharyngeal accumulations of mucus, saliva, CSF and blood, particularly common in maxillo-facial injuries, are readily inhaled, as are vomited stomach contents. Treatment properly begins at the scene of the accident, and most ambulance crews and first-aid workers have been instructed in the correct emergency positioning of an unconscious patient, i.e. the lateral or even the face down position, but this is a measure to be taken only in the absence of proper facilities. If the airway can be maintained then the supine position is by far the best for the normal respiratory movements of the chest.

Once in hospital, and with the proper equipment to hand, pharyngeal suction should be performed immediately if seen to be necessary, and an oral airway then introduced. There should be no hesitation in intubating the trachea if the airway can be more satisfactorily maintained in this way, and endotracheal intubation becomes essential if there are chest injuries causing respiratory inadequacy. When intubation is obviously necessary but difficult to perform because of extreme restlessness or decerebrate spasms there is no contraindication to giving a drug such as Droperidol to quieten the patient for a short while. The noisy struggling unco-operative patient with cerebral and maybe other injuries derives no benefit from being allowed to continue in this state.

180

Intubation and Tracheostomy. Every doctor working in a casualty department or an intensive care unit should be able to perform endo-tracheal intubation. Tracheostomy, on the other hand, should hardly ever be necessary as an emergency procedure in a hospital, especially where head injuries are concerned. It should always be an elective procedure done by a trained surgeon with the facilities that only an operating theatre can ensure. No surgeon would care to undertake this operation outside of a theatre, particularly on a patient who is probably cyanosed and has gross venous congestion. Therefore no one can reasonably expect a junior doctor to attempt such a procedure. For him to do so, when intubation would be just as effective, would be reprehensible.

In most instances, after a few days of endo-tracheal intubation, the need for continuing artificial maintenance of the airway resolves itself. Bleeding has invariably ceased, mucosal hypersecretion has abated and only very rarely is continuing CSF leakage so copious as to constitute a problem to airway patency. Even amongst those patients who have not yet regained consciousness many are much lighter and their cough reflexes have returned. There is, however, a very definite place for tracheostomy, particularly in patients with severe maxillo-facial injuries. Strangely enough, although too often this operation is done unnecessarily, when it is indicated it is often done too late. In most cases its necessity should be anticipated and the operation performed 24 hours before its need becomes really obvious. The creation of a tracheostomy brings its own peculiar problems, notably infection or the possibility of subsequent airway stenosis. The latter in itself is sufficient reason for leaving this operation to those who are accustomed to the procedure. The rule in an emergency should be:

INTUBATE IMMEDIATELY AND THEN CONSIDER TRACHEOSTOMY AT LEISURE

Artificial Ventilation. Skilfully managed artificial ventilation can be of great value in helping to tide over the period of inefficient respiration due to raised intracranial pressure or chest injuries. It is not intended to enter into a discussion on the methods of ventilation, this having been dealt with in Chapter 2. However, a

181

very real problem arises in the case of the deteriorating brain-injured patient who has a sudden respiratory arrest and develops dilated and fixed pupils. He is often immediately intubated, coupled up to a ventilator, and with this form of respiration his heart action continues normally, his colour remains good, but the pupils remain unaltered. The question then arises as to how long one should persist. In our experience, to continue for more than six hours, during which time all attempts to reduce intra-cranial tension have produced no improvement, is futile. Probably the only time that such measures are successful is when the arrest takes place just before an operation is about to be performed which relieves increasing intracranial pressure from haemorrhage or other cause. The only justification for con-tinuing artificial respiration beyond six hours is if the patient is a potential donor of kidneys or other organs for transplantation.

Ideally, the use of an artificial ventilator should be carefully monitored by estimating blood oxygen and carbon dioxide levels. This is not always possible, and a very common fault in the use of respirators is to unwittingly hyperventilate the patient. When disconnecting a patient from the respirator to see if spontaneous breathing has returned it is advisable to wait for upwards of six to eight minutes, to be certain that continued cessation of respiration is not the result of extreme alkalosis. Trial disconnection might advantageously be preceded by reducing the minute volume for a short while so that the CO_2 level of the blood can rise sufficiently to stimulate the onset of respiration.

Cerebral Death. The increasing use of tissue transplantation has led to a great deal of critical appraisal of what constitutes death. Not all organs or systems cease to function at the same moment, but the real difficulty arises in the fact that cases have been reported of one or two patients recovering after apparently complete cessation of CNS function, particularly as evidenced by electrical silence on the EEG recordings. Such cases, however, seem to be extremely rare when one considers the large number of deaths which take place from brain injuries. In practice, death can be assumed to have taken place when there has been spontaneous respiratory arrest and no evidence of a reversal of this state of affairs despite immediate and adequate artificial ventilation together with treatment of the cerebral injury. It is reasonable to wait up to six hours for signs of recovery, but if none have appeared at the end of this time it is almost certain that they never will. The persistence of dilated fixed pupils, a progressive drying and clouding of the cornea, a steadily falling blood pressure and signs of peripheral circulatory failure can leave none but the most enthusiastic in any doubt that the situation is hopeless.

Circulatory State. When the urgent respiratory problems have been dealt with attention should then be turned to the state of the patient's circulation. For all practical purposes haemorrhagic shock is never the result of a head injury alone. If it is present in an unconscious patient a very careful examination should be made for internal haemorrhage, e.g. a ruptured spleen, if no other source of blood loss is apparent. When cerebral trauma is part of a multiple injuries complex and the total blood loss has been large, transfusion with whole blood as soon as possible is an important part of treatment. The oxygen carrying capacity of the blood in the cerebral circulation is, within limits, far more important than the pressure at which the blood is flowing.

Assessment of CNS Injury

This should only be carried out when any respiratory deficits and the grosser degrees of blood loss have been corrected.

In these patients there can be a bewildering array of abnormal neurological signs, some of which defy interpretation by even the most experienced neurologists. Fortunately, the object of examination in the early stages following injury is not to study the minutiae but to assess the over-all function of the nervous system, particularly with regard to consciousness, and to follow the patient's progress in the subsequent hours to detect any signs of deterioration; the latter could be due to an eminently treatable lesion. In order to do this it is necessary to concentrate on certain clinical features only:

1. The level of consciousness.
2. The state of the pupils.
3. The vital functions, i.e. respiration, pulse rate, blood pressure.

4. External signs of potentially dangerous skull fractures.

5. Signs of a hemiplegia.

These features are listed more or less in order of priority; certainly the level of consciousness comes first and is by far the most important.

IT MUST ALWAYS BE AGAINST THE BACKGROUND OF THE CONSCIOUS LEVEL THAT ALL OTHER SIGNS ARE JUDGED

It is worth repeating that it is in the first eight hours from the time of injury that the more urgent intracranial complications, especially extra-dural haemorrhage, will develop and, to detect them early, frequent, regular and accurate assessments are essential throughout this period. The failure to observe regularly is probably a commoner cause of unnecessary death from head injuries than a lack of diagnostic skill.

Charts and Charting. A chart of some sort is required for recording purposes,and, unfortunately, there is no agreed standard pattern. Some are so complicated and cater for such a mass of detail that the advantage of an instant pictorial representation of the patient's state and progress is lost. Unless a chart has been specifically designed for research purposes it should record only essential information and, by employing symbols rather than words, be capable of giving an instant picture of the patient's course. More often than not these early observations and chartings are carried out by nurses, and it is important that they should know exactly what they are looking for and how to record their findings. It is so often the case that they are asked for too many observations, too frequently and over too long a period. This leads inevitably to an inaccurate and unreliable record. It is also important to ensure that the nursing staff know when to report as well as record significant changes. A fall in conscious level, the dilatation of one pupil or the onset of irregular breathing should be notified immediately, as should also any profound change in heart rate or the blood pressure. More gradual changes in the latter two functions are usually only of significance, assuming the patient's conscious level is satisfactory, if the trend of the deviation persists for three successive quarter-hourly observations.

184

How we have attempted to meet these requirements is detailed later as each feature is discussed. The time sequence for recordings starts with the estimated time of the injury and the first assessment appears after an appropriate interval along the time base. Our charts (Fig. 6.2) are designed on 0·5 cm squared paper and cater for:

1. Time.
2. Respiratory rate.
3. Pulse rate.
4. Blood pressure.
5. State of pupils.
6. Temperature.
7. Conscious level.

During the first eight hours following the injury we routinely observe the patient at least every half an hour; quarter-hourly if there is obvious cause for concern. Thereafter the intervals are lengthened, considerably so if the patient is now conscious. A planned system of reducing the frequency and extent of observations can appreciably lighten the load on both the nursing staff and the patient. Particularly in children, nothing can be more conducive to so-called cerebral irritation than being disturbed every fifteen minutes throughout the night to have a light shone in one's eyes.

1. *Level of Consciousness.* Our practice is to recognize five levels of consciousness, and the majority of patients can be readily placed into one of these groups without much difficulty. The level assessed is recorded on the chart as a number within the range 1 to 5.

1. Fully conscious, orientated and rational.
2. Conscious but drowsy or confused. Speaking and/or obeying commands accordingly.
3. Unconscious but responding to pain with purposeful (flexion) movements of the limbs and, maybe, vocalizing.
4. Unconscious but responding to pain with reflex non-purposeful (extensor) movements of the limbs, the state of so-called 'decerebrate rigidity'.
5. Unconscious and with no appreciable response to pain.

The Painful Stimulus. A number of methods of applying such

NEUROLOGICAL OBSERVATIONS CHART

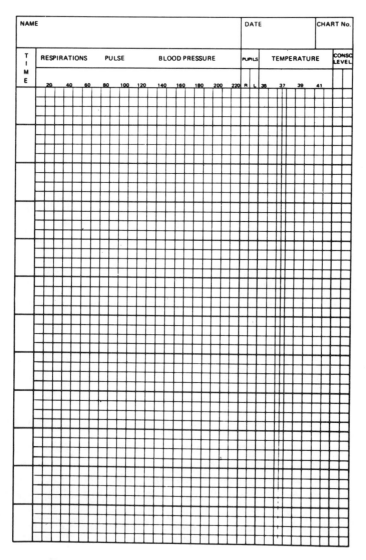

Fig. 6.2.

a stimulus are in use but many of them are ineffective or unneccessarily traumatic. There is no place for nipping and twisting the patient's skin thus leaving his limbs covered in bruises. The easiest, and one of the most consistently effective no matter who applies it, is to rub hard over the manubrium sterni with the knuckles. A fairly uniform degree of stimulus which is certainly painful and response evoking is thereby obtained. It goes without saying that it is not necessary to apply this stimulus to patients in conscious levels 1 or 2.

2. *State of Pupils.* The range of possible pupil sizes, shapes and reactions is wide, and this frequently leads to some confusion amongst observers as well as inconsistency in charting. The points of particular importance to be noted are:

(a) The size of each pupil.

In practice we have found that it is sufficient to record pupil size as large or dilated, average or normal, small or constricted. These are shown respectively and pictorially on the charts as a circle completely occupying the square, a circle within the square, or a central solid dot (Fig. 6.3).

(b) The reaction to light of each pupil.

The reaction of the pupil to light is shown by placing a + sign within the circle; absence of reaction is denoted by a − sign. The constricted pupil, denoted by a solid dot, is already in the reactive state and therefore its ability to react to light is implied. A not uncommon mistake is to shine the light across the eye rather than directly into the eye; this frequently leads to the reporting of a non-reacting pupil. A sluggish reaction is of no great clinical significance and, moreover, its presence is often a matter of opinion. For all practical purposes a pupil either reacts or it does not, the speed of reaction being irrelevant. The shape of the pupil is likewise of no immediate clinical value.

As mentioned above pupillary abnormalities must always be considered against the level of consciousness. The finding of a unilateral dilated non-reacting pupil in a fully conscious patient certainly implies nerve injury, but it is not the result of III nerve compression by uncal herniation.

3. *Vital Functions.* These are all liable to be adversely affected by rising intracranial pressure; the heart rate slows, the blood

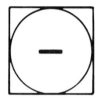 = **Dilated and non-reacting**

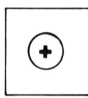 = **Normal and reacting**

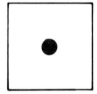 = **Constricted**

Fig. 6.3.

pressure rises and breathing becomes irregular. Before these changes are really noticeable, however, the level of consciousness will either have fallen or have been very low all along. It is not uncommon in healthy patients, particularly young men, who are conscious and obviously recovering from their injuries to find a pulse rate of 40–50 per minute. In these circumstances the bradycardia is no cause for alarm. On the other hand, if the patient has been deeply unconscious from the start these changes in respiration and circulation become the only indications of a worsening condition.

4. *External Signs of Potentially Dangerous Skull Fractures.* These signs can be of great diagnostic significance and their presence should always be looked for and recorded at the earliest possible moment.

A boggy swelling in the temporal region should be taken as indicating the possibility of an underlying fracture of the

188

temporal bone and a co-existing extra-dural haemorrhage. If the patient is unconscious, has a dilated fixed pupil on the same side as the swelling and a contra-lateral hemiplegia the possibility becomes a probability and no time should be lost in preparing for an immediate operation.

Bleeding from the external auditory canal or the nose, sub-conjunctival haemorrhage and periorbital haematoma all suggest the presence of a fractured base of skull with the possibility of correspondingly severe cerebral injuries. It has already been mentioned that when the victim was wearing a crash helmet at the time of the accident there may be very little external evidence to hint at the severe intracranial injuries that might be present.

5. *Hemiplegia.* Even when the patient is unconscious the presence of hemiplegia is usually easily recognized by the absence of spontaneous or reflex movements on the affected side. It might be present from the outset but its first appearance a few hours after the injury indicates a progressive lesion of the contralateral hemisphere and could signify the accumulation of a compressing extracerebral haematoma, although the cause will most often prove to be cortical contusion or oedema. Occasionally a unilateral subdural haematoma produces an ipsi-lateral hemiplegia; this is due to a displacement of the cerebral hemisphere and brain stem to the opposite side and the contra-lateral crus cerebrum then impacts against the margin of the tentorium.

Some Special Aspects of Head Injury Management

The X-ray Examination of Head Injuries. The implications of the term 'fractured skull' should be kept in perspective. To the lay person it invariably means a serious head injury, but, medically, this is by no means always the case. Severe brain injury might be unaccompanied by a fracture of the skull; alternatively, extensive fractures of the vault might be associated with only minimal brain damage. If they are to be of diagnostic value, whenever possible films should be taken with a proper skull unit apparatus. Portable X-rays are frequently of poor quality so far as the skull detail is concerned, but there are

189

occasions when, because of urgency or the restrictions imposed by associated injuries, they are the only practicable means of obtaining the necessary information.

Somehow it has become virtually a ritual to X-ray all cases of head injury, but it is our belief that this examination can be safely and properly omitted in the majority of patients. This majority consists of all those patients who have, as the result of a blow to the head, sustained minor concussion from which they show every indication of recovering rapidly. As indicated earlier the correct management of such patients is to admit and observe them until the danger period is over; the presence of a simple linear fracture of the vault should make no difference to the management of these cases and there are certainly no special measures to be taken once the observation period is over. Of course, those patients who show signs of a greater degree of damage to the brain or have external evidence of possible skull injuries must be X-rayed, but this examination always should be done on the basis of clinical indications and not because the doctor feels, mistakenly as it happens, that he is under a legal obligation to do so. This might be controversial advice, but it serves to place the emphasis on clinical judgement and a planned procedure. We have followed this practice now for more than five years, during which time a large number of head injuries have been seen, and nothing has happened to make us change our views. The greatest mistake of all is to send home prematurely the 'recovering patient' because his skull X-ray showed no evidence of a fracture.

An all too common fault in practice is to request X-ray examination when the patient is in no fit state to have this carried out, either successfully or safely. To attempt to obtain films of diagnostic value on a patient who is restless and unco-operative is futile; to send the patient to the X-ray department when he is in need of resuscitation is reprehensible. Time should never be wasted in diverting to the X-ray department the patient who is deteriorating rapidly and who should be on his way to the operating theatre.

The Treatment of Decerebrate Rigidity. This, as is the case with concussion, is another well-recognized clinical phenomenon about which there is considerable doubt and debate as to its

physio-pathological basis. In its commonest form the patient is
unconscious and responds to painful stimulation, or even irritation of his air passages, by extension spasms in all limbs together
with fist clenching and pronation in the arms and plantar flexion
of the feet. Such paroxysms of activity may arise apparently
spontaneously without any form of precipitating stimulation. At
times they may be seen to occur asymmetrically or to alternate
with some flexion movements of the limbs. The most favoured
explanation of this state is that there is disturbed function at
brain-stem level, possibly affecting both the reticular formations
and cerebellar mechanisms, but nothing more specific than this
can be said.

It is undesirable to allow repeated frequent paroxysms to occur,
as they inferfere noticeably with regular respiratory movements
and can lead to a rising body temperature as a result of the greatly
increased metabolic heat production in the affected muscles.
This tendency to pyrexia might also in part be due to injury to
heat regulating mechanisms mediated in the diencephalon.
Hyperpyrexia can quickly develop and become a dangerous and
worrying feature of this condition.

The most effective treatment available is to give small but
regular doses of Pethidine and chlorpromazine intramuscularly.
In an adult 25 mgm of each is an average effective dose, but this
can be increased or reduced according to the patient's response.
In children the dose is determined correspondingly by the body
weight, but again it can be varied depending upon the response.
At the same time the body temperature should be carefully
watched and, in all cases, monitored by a constant rectal recording. Axillary or other skin temperatures are completely
unreliable for this purpose. If the temperature is rising despite
the administration of drugs, active cooling by means of wet
sponging and the use of electric fans should be instituted.

The Treatment of Cerebral Oedema. It is well recognized that
dangerously high levels of raised intracranial pressure can result
from traumatic cerebral oedema alone and in the absence of
space occupying haemorrhage. This form of cerebral oedema is
a subject which has of late given rise to considerable interest,
and in several neurosurgical centres much research into this
problem is being carried out. However, at the present time there

191

is very little known of the mechanisms involved which result in this state developing. One of the main practical problems is differentiating this cause of raised intracranial pressure from haemorrhage. Cerebral angiography or echo-encephalography can be helpful in arriving at a correct diagnosis, but these are investigations which can only be carried out in a special centre and the results are not always completely reliable. In an emergency situation, when all the signs indicate that the intracranial pressure is steadily rising, an attempt must be made to reverse this trend whatever its cause.

First and foremost in treatment is endotracheal intubation together with controlled and moderate hyperventilation. By reducing CO_2 levels and cerebral venous pressure this form of treatment can play a major part in combating progressive oedema.

So-called 'brain shrinking' solutions, which work on the basis of increasing the osmotic pressure of the blood and thus reducing tissue fluid volume, are available for intravenous use; an example is Mannitol 25%. They are very effective but must be used with caution, for if given too quickly they lead to a rapid increase in the total circulating blood volume with an accompanying peripheral vasodilatation to accommodate this extra load. This vasodilatation can in turn lead to renewed haemorrhage at the site of any blood vessel trauma. If intracranial in situation this renewed haemorrhage now takes place even more readily because of the concomitant reduction in brain volume. Where the possibility of intracranial vascular damage exists it is recommended that the solution be given no faster than 50 ml per hour, although the first 50 ml can be given within the space of 5—10 minutes.

A third method advocated for the reduction of cerebral oedema is the administration of steroids, such as dexamethasone or betamethasone, in doses which are both enormous and quite unphysiological. The usual dose, given intramuscularly, is an initial one of 10 mg which is followed by 5 mg every six hours. Certainly such treatment can have an impressive and remarkably beneficial effect in the oedema accompanying cerebral tumours, but the author has been disappointed with their use in traumatic oedema. Even so they should be given a trial if the situation demands.

Head Injuries in Children. The reaction displayed by a child to a head injury is often strikingly different to that seen in an adult, and in no other age group does one so frequently see such a surprising discrepancy between the apparent severity of the injuring forces and the relative mildness of the brain damage inflicted. Falls of 15—20 feet or more from upper storey windows are not uncommonly the cause of only a moderate degree of concussion. And yet, whilst this concussion state is present, the clinical picture to the inexperienced observer can be quite alarming and prolonged. For some hours the child is often drowsy and, when roused, exhibits obvious irritability. This state might persist for a day or two to be followed by a similar period of lethargy and occasional vomiting, but complete recovery almost invariably takes place within a few days.

Whilst considering head injuries in children an important point must be mentioned with regard to the 'battered baby' with head injuries. In these children sub-galeal and sub-dural haemorrhages are fairly common, and the total loss of blood from the circulation at both these sites and elsewhere in the body can result in a severe loss of circulatory volume and haemoglobin. In such cases the possibility of a blood transfusion in emergency treatment should always be considered; it is one of the few instances in which a head injury alone can cause haemorrhagic shock.

Treatment of Co-existing Injuries. 'When can we go ahead and deal with the patient's other injuries?' is a question which is often asked, especially when the treatment of these injuries requires an anaesthetic. The answer must always be determined by weighing the gravity and urgency of these injuries against the state of the brain. When serious internal haemorrhage or thoracic injuries demand immediate operative treatment they must take absolute priority for obvious reasons. On the other hand if the treatment of the associated injuries is not immediately necessary then it is preferable to allow at least six hours to elapse from the time of injury during which the need for any neurosurgical intervention can be ascertained. Whatever decision is reached, either to treat immediately or after an interval, the special requirements of the brain-injured patient are always the same; a skilful anaesthetic technique with the prompt replacement of any

193

blood loss. Anoxia, hypercapnia and hypotension must never be allowed to complicate the treatment of other injuries when the brain is already in jeopardy. Even when the patient is so deeply unconscious as to not require an anaesthetic it is important to intubate and connect him to an anaesthetic machine supplying oxygen and thereby ensure adequate pulmonary ventilation. It is by no means uncommon for a patient not so treated to have his face inadvertently covered with operating towels and be re-breathing the same air with all the consequent adverse effects.

The Relief of Pain. Fortunately it is not very often that this is a problem in the management of head injuries. When it does arise it is usually in the case of the patient with a very mild head injury but with more serious painful lesions elsewhere. If there are no signs of brain injury of any consequence, or possible complications, we have no hesitation in giving Pethidine 50 mgm which is sufficient to afford a little relief without any significant depressant effect on the CNS. If there are any persisting signs of brain injury however, no analgesic drugs should be given in the first six hours following injury; thereafter the case is decided by the patient's condition and progress. In practice, those patients for whom such drugs are contraindicated rarely require them.

Post-concussional Confusion. It is worth bearing in mind that the mental after-effects of moderate to severe concussion, for memory and orientation in particular, usually persist for a longer period than the superficial behaviour of the patient would suggest. He might seem to answer questions, talk to his visitors and read newspapers quite normally and yet subsequently have no recollection of these incidents. Careful observation will often reveal evidence of this incomplete recovery if the possibility is borne in mind. An extra day or two in hospital or a forewarning to his relatives before his discharge will prevent distress and criticism.

CEREBRAL TUMOUR

Every now and then a patient with a cerebral tumour presents urgently with a short history of headache, vomiting, maybe neurological deficits and a quickly deteriorating level of consciousness. The illness might have started only a few days previously but relatives often relate a preceding period of vague ill-health, the true cause of which was far from obvious. Probably many cerebral tumours have a lengthy initial silent phase during which time the brain accommodates the enlarging growth by a combination of gradual displacement and compression. Eventually a stage is reached where the local distortion produces venous embarrassment and the space occupying effect is then quickly augmented by oedema, both in the tumour and in the surrounding brain tissue, with the production of the first real symptoms and signs of the disease. This breakdown in adaptation, as well as occurring at a critical size of tumour growth, might also be precipitated by the disturbance of an otherwise minor head injury or a lumbar puncture unwisely performed on a patient undergoing investigations for seemingly vague cerebral illness such as confusion and headaches. For obvious reasons it is important to be on the look-out for cases presenting after injury. There is nearly always an interval of a few days between the accident and the patient arriving at the hospital. Papilloedema is usually obvious by this stage and provides the essential clue to the correct diagnosis.

In this situation the most effective treatment available is the administration of beta-methasone or dexa-methoasone. An initial dose, given by intra-muscular injection, of 10 mg, followed every six hours by doses of 5 mg can produce a remarkable reversal of the patient's condition. Within twelve to eighteen hours of starting treatment the patient, who might have been unconscious and hemiplegic, can be sitting up, talking and now showing either no paralysis or only a mild paresis. This early beneficial effect of steroids is almost certainly brought about by a reduction of the fluid content of the tumour area rather than an anti-neoplastic action. They can undoubtedly exert the latter effect on many tumours, and not only those of the brain, but it probably takes at least several days for this action to get under way.

If the patient's condition is critical when he is first seen, endo-tracheal intubation followed by a short period of moderate hyperventilation is often successful in bringing about an improvement, but it is an effect which is not easy to maintain and hyperventilation can only be used for a limited period. The

195

intravenous infusion of 25% Mannitol is also useful for urgent resuscitation but, in both cases, their subsequent early replacement by steroid therapy is necessary.

Posterior fossa tumours, by obstructing the aqueduct or the IV ventricle, not infrequently produce acute severe rises in intracranial pressure. The diagnosis is seldom in doubt; severe headache, occipital pain and maybe some neck rigidity, papilloedema and signs of cerebellar dysfunction or cranial nerve lesions are usually present. From time to time a patient will present with repeated transient attacks of loss of consciousness and apnoea. The relief of CSF pressure is a matter of urgency and, unless the patient can be speedily transferred to a neurosurgical unit, tapping of the lateral ventricle must be carried out.

A burr hole is made 3 cm to the right of the sagittal line and 14 cm behind the nasion. A small hole is made, by diathermy, through the dura mater and, through this hole, a brain cannula or a lumbar puncture needle is introduced into the lateral ventricle. The needle is kept in the coronal plane but is directed medially, aiming for the A—P axis of the nasion. The ventricle in these patients is usually enlarged and is not difficult to locate at a depth of about 4—5 cm below the dura. After releasing the pressure a No. 3 soft rubber catheter can be used in place of the needle and indwelling drainage continued whilst the patient is transferred.

SUB-ARACHNOID HAEMORRHAGE

There is rarely any doubt about the diagnosis in this condition. The sudden onset of severe headache, with or without loss of consciousness a few minutes later, is characteristic. Vomiting is common and neck stiffness is usually very evident. Hypertension is a frequent finding, but it is more often reactive to the haemorrhage than essential in nature. It is our practice not to treat hypertension in this phase of the illness.

Early treatment should be carried out in whichever hospital the patient is taken to and long journeys to a neurological centre can be harmful at this stage. There is almost never any indication or justification for either angiography or surgery in the first two or three days. During this period management is directed towards confirming the diagnosis by lumbar puncture and then controlling headache and restlessness by the use of Pethidine and chlorpromazine.

Attitudes to the role of surgery in the treatment of the cause of the haemorrhage vary but where such treatment is favoured the object of surgery is to prevent further haemorrhage in the patient who is recovering from the first onslaught. Cerebral angiography should be regarded as a pre-operative investigation and, as such, should be considered only when the patient is well enough to undergo any surgical procedure that might be indicated. There is no place for angiography in the deeply unconscious patient. Also, it should not be performed on the patient who remains drowsy, has persisting severe headache and in whom neck rigidity is very evident. In these patients arterial spasm is almost certainly present and angiography not only fails to show an aneurysm but can adversely affect the patient's condition.

A recurrence of haemorrhage is usually evident from a sudden worsening of headache, a fall in conscious level, or elevation of the blood pressure. However it is not uncommon to encounter patients in whom there is a gradual increase in the severity of the headache and who slowly become more drowsy and less responsive. Quite often this gradual deterioration over two or three days is due not to a vascular cause but to obstruction to the extra-cerebral CSF circulation by blood which has entered the basal cisterns. In these circumstances a slow drainage lumbar puncture, removing some 30 ml of fluid after confirming the high pressure, will bring about a dramatic improvement. This might have to be repeated several times, at intervals of a few days, until normal conditions are restored.

Chapter 7

Shock

HEDLEY BERRY

CLASSIFICATION

Cardiogenic

Peripheral Circulatory Failure:

Hypovolaemic Shock
Bacteraemic Shock

PATHOPHYSIOLOGY

Changes in: Microcirculation
Blood
Pulmonary Function
Cardiac Function

CLINICAL SIGNS

MONITORING THE SHOCKED PATIENT

Fluid Deficit:

Haematocrit
Blood Volume
ECF Volume
CVP

Efficiency of the Pumping Mechanism:

Heart and BP
Renal Function
Cardiac Output

MANAGEMENT AND THERAPY

Respiratory Function

IV Fluids:

Volume Replacement
Type of Fluid

Acidosis

Bacteraemic Shock:

Antibiotics
Steroids
Surgery

Vaso-active Drugs

Cardiac Glycosides

No single definition of the word 'shock' can include all the complex underlying mechanisms which may exist, but it is probably most satisfactory to regard 'shock' as a clinical syndrome which results from an acute decrease in the oxygen delivery to the vital tissues of the body. Every patient who becomes shocked can be said to be suffering from a failure of tissue perfusion and tissue anoxia which produces the syndrome of pallor, sweating brow, rapid thready pulse, cold cyanosed extremities and usually hypotension which the clinician should instantly recognize.

Although the resulting clinical picture may be very similar whatever the cause of the shocked state, the exact mechanisms whereby tissue perfusion is reduced will differ from patient to patient, depending on the underlying cause of the shock. The modern intensive care unit, with its facilities for monitoring and treating shocked patients has done much to clarify these differences in the pathological and physiological problems posed. Only if the clinician has an understanding of these problems can treatment be carried out on a rational basis and a consistently successful outcome expected. In many shocked patients the diagnosis may not always be apparent and treatment may have to be commenced before an accurate diagnosis is made. Under these circumstances it is essential that a broad classification of the possible underlying factors is borne in mind, so that the mechanisms responsible are clarified and accurate therapy instituted without delay.

CLASSIFICATION

The underlying causes of the shock syndrome may be considered under two main headings: cardiogenic shock in which the venous return of blood to the heart is adequate but there is a failure of the pump itself or an obstruction to its outflow, and peripheral circulatory failure when the main pathophysiological changes occur in the arterioles and capillaries of the peripheral microcirculation.

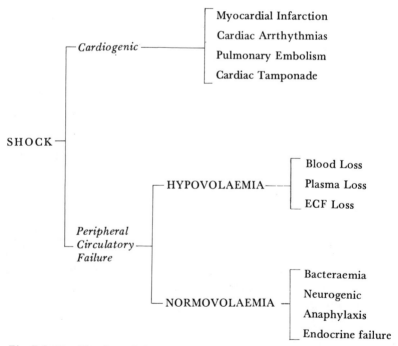

Fig. 7.1. Classification of shock.

Shock

Cardiogenic Shock is fully discussed in Chapter 1 to which the reader is referred for details of its causes and management. In the present context it should be remembered however, that whatever the main precipitating cause of shock may be, cardiac failure due to ischaemia, infarction or arrhythmias may play a significant role in the clinical picture, especially in the elderly. Similarly, cardiac tamponade due to a haemopericardium should always be considered in a patient suffering from multiple injuries which involve the chest. Included under the heading of cardiogenic shock is pulmonary embolism, which often presents a problem in differential diagnosis, particularly in the patient who becomes shocked post-operatively. In cardiogenic shock the venous return to the heart is adequate to fill the pump and this is reflected in the raised central venous pressure, measured close to the heart in the superior or inferior venae cavae.

In contrast, the central venous pressure is not raised, and is commonly lowered, in peripheral circulatory failure. This may occur because of a reduction in the volume of circulatory blood (hypovolaemia) or because of an abnormal vasodilatation occurring in the capillary or arteriolar beds resulting in pooling of blood, which is, in effect, lost to the circulation (normovolaemic shock).

Hypovolaemia may result from a loss of whole blood, plasma or extracellular fluid from the circulation. A reduction in the amount of blood in the circulation is the most frequent serious effect of traumatic shock, which can be defined as shock following injury. The patient admitted to the intensive care unit with multiple injuries following, for example, a road traffic accident can present some of the most difficult problems in management and resuscitation, and it is in estimating the volume of blood that the patient has lost that errors commonly arise. Too great an emphasis can be placed in the patient's pulse, blood pressure and skin colour as the indices of shock necessitating the need for transfusion. It must be remembered that a young adult may lose as much as 25% of his blood volume and yet have only a mild tachycardia and a blood pressure within the normal range. Although such a patient may not be in need of urgent transfusion, further haemorrhage, or continued concealed bleeding may result in a sudden and precipitous fall in blood pressure. The patient who presents with a tachycardia, hypotension and

201

a pale, cold sweating skin will obviously require transfusion to make good the deficit which may amount to as much as 40% of his blood volume.

In the case of an open wound, some estimate of the blood loss may be made from the size of the wound and visible blood shed. When the blood loss is concealed however, estimation is often more difficult. Hidden loss after bone injuries, particulary with fractures of the femur, spine and pelvis with retroperitoneal haematomas often escape recognition. It has been estimated that injured tissue the size of a fist represents a loss of approximately half a litre of blood. A fractured shaft of femur with visible swelling of the thigh will have lost as much as two litres of blood into the tissues. It is sometimes difficult to distinguish deformity from tissue swelling but the extent of radiological deformity will usually give some guide. Any fracture of any bone site may contain as much as one litre of blood and multiple fractures always require correction of hypovolaemia.

The greatest difficulty in assessing blood loss arises when the injury involves the trunk. In chest injuries, blood lost into the pleural cavity is frequently underestimated and not recognized because the clinical signs of fluid in the pleural cavity are difficult or impossible to elicit in the injured patient, and radiological signs may not be evident until a litre or more of blood has been lost. The possibility that such a loss has occurred should always be borne in mind in multiple injuries which include fracture of ribs.

Extensive blood loss due to intra-abdominal injury, most commonly due to rupture of the spleen or liver, will produce the signs of peritoneal irritation, which demand immediate attention. When intraperitoneal haemorrhage complicates a multiple injury, however, especially involving the chest and spine, muscle spasm in the abdominal wall may completely mask the signs of abdominal injury, so that they are easily missed in the early stages. Under these circumstances, when the patient has obviously lost blood which cannot otherwise be accounted for, a peritoneal 'tap' may be invaluable in deciding if intra-abdominal bleeding has occurred. A fine bore needle is inserted into the peritoneal cavity, through all four quadrants of the abdominal wall in turn, and aspirated with a syringe to detect the presence of blood.

Shock

Hypovolaemia due predominantly to a loss of plasma is a problem encountered mainly in the management of the severely burned patient. Many litres of plasma, in addition to other intravenous fluids may be required in the resuscitation of such a patient, the details of which are beyond the scope of this chapter. A plasma deficit may also contribute to shock accompanying such conditions as a strangulated bowel obstruction and acute pancreatitis.

Shock due to a deficit of extracellular fluid results from abnormal losses from the gastro-intestinal tract. The loss may be obvious as in the patient who suffers from copious vomiting, severe diarrhoea or an external fistula, or it may be concealed in the lumen of the gut. It is often forgotten that in a case of advanced intestinal obstruction as much as four litres of fluid may be aspirated and much more left behind in the so-called 'third space' of the gut lumen. This represents approximately one-tenth of the total body water and one-third of the extracellular fluid volume, containing up to 120 mEq/litre of Na^+ and 14 mEq/litre of K^+. Such a patient's hypovolaemic shock will only be corrected when this large deficit is made good.

Bacteraemia follows myocardial infarction and trauma as a common cause of shock in hospital patients. The incidence of shock in patients who develop bacteraemia is impossible to estimate accurately, since in so many patients a bacteraemia is transient and unrecognized. It has been estimated that between 20 and 40 per cent of bacteraemic patients become shocked, and in this group the mortality remains extremely high, varying in different series from 30 to 80 per cent. Bacteraemia is therefore a very important contributory factor in the death of many hospital patients. In some reported series the incidence of bacteraemic shock has increased by as much as ten-fold during the past 20 years. There are probably several reasons for this. Certainly a greater awareness of the importance of bacteraemia has led to the diagnosis being made more frequently. The increasing use of antibiotics has resulted in the emergence of resistant strains of bacteria and therefore an increased likelihood of bacteraemia occurring. The use of prophylactic antibiotics, particularly in abdominal surgery has also been incriminated. In early life the majority of cases occur in the neonatal period and

203

in later life the incidence rises sharply with age. The increasing age of the hospital population may therefore contribute to the rising frequency of bacteraemic shock.

A precipitating cause for bacteraemic shock can usually be found on enquiring into the patient's recent history. In elderly males, operations or manipulations on the urinary tract in the presence of urinary infection is probably the most common cause of bacteraemia. Pelvic surgery, childbearing and septic abortions are responsible for the increased incidence in young females. In abdominal surgery, peritonitis, wound infections and biliary infections feature high in the list of underlying causes. The possible introduction of bacteria into the blood stream from an intravenous infusion should always be considered when no other obvious cause is apparent. Debilitated patients suffering from malignant disease, blood dyscrasias, hepatic cirrhosis or diabetes mellitus are particularly prone to bacteraemia, as are patients taking corticosteroids and cytotoxic agents.

When no obvious underlying cause is apparent, bacteraemia must be considered as an aetiological factor in any patient who becomes shocked. If the diagnosis is suspected blood must immediately be taken for culture, so that the infecting organism and its sensitivity to antibiotics can be determined as soon as possible. Since a fatal outcome may be rapid, however, treatment must be started before the results of culture are available. Gram negative and gram positive organisms may both be responsible for bacteraemic shock and a good guide may be obtained from previous cultures taken from a wound, peritoneal pus or urine. Strains of Escherichia coli are the commonest agents, with Aerobacter, Proteus and Pseudomonas, next in order of frequency.

Endocrine failure presenting with the shock syndrome is most commonly encountered as adrenal insufficiency. This is particularly relevant in the intensive care unit when a patient becomes shocked after major surgery or trauma and the possibility that the patient was taking corticosteroids for some unrelated condition has been overlooked. Enquiries should always be made about previous steroid therapy and the patient supported postoperatively by adrenocortical hormone therapy when necessary.

Neurogenic shock may occur after a severe spinal injury when

sympathetic paralysis results in capillary and arteriolar vasodilatation and pooling of blood in the peripheral circulation,
producing, in effect, a hypovolaemic shock. Anaphylaxis is
included to complete the list of possible aetiological factors in
shock although it is seldom a problem encountered in the
intensive care unit and the clinical picture which follows the
administration of an allergen should be easily recognized.

It must be remembered that the shocked patient often
presents a complicated picture and the clinical state can seldom
be attributed to any single one of the possible aetiological
factors. The elderly patient who becomes shocked following
operation for strangulated intestinal obstruction may have a
plasma and extracellular fluid deficit if replacement has been
inadequate, and the blood lost into the bowel and at operation
may have been underestimated. In addition, bacteraemia may
have occurred, and an element of cardiac failure can also complicate the clinical picture. Such patients require full and careful
assessment and successful treatment can only be based on a
knowledge of the pathophysiological changes which occur
throughout the body.

PATHOPHYSIOLOGY

From such studies as are now possible in the modern intensive
care unit, much has been learnt in recent years about the
changes which occur in shock. A full evaluation however, of
treatment in clinical shock is difficult because it is rare to find
comparable injuries in comparable patients and investigation of
patients must necessarily be overshadowed by their treatment.
Much of the information upon which treatment is based is, therefore, derived from experiments on animals. This has the disadvantage that species differences occur and the responses of an
animal to a shock pathogen may be very different to the human
response. Indeed, it was from animal experiments, that the term
irreversible shock was first coined. The term irreversible shock
should be abandoned in clinical practice, for it implies that as
shock progresses a point comes beyond which recovery is impossible and death is inevitable. Refractory shock probably
describes better the patients who do not respond to initial treatment, a term which implies that modification in management is

required, since many cases are in fact instances of unrecognized myocardial failure, inadequate fluid replacement and septicaemia.

Microcirculatory Changes

Fig. 7.2 diagrammatically represents the changes which can occur in the microcirculation of the shocked patient.

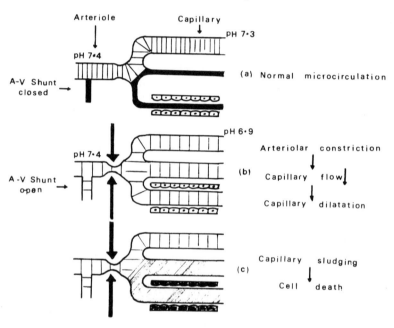

Fig. 7.2. Microcirculatory changes in shock (after Hardaway 1965).

In the normal state of affairs (Fig. 7.2(a)), only about one-third of the capillaries are perfused at any one time, while the others are resting until they open in rotation in response to the metabolic needs of the cells adjacent to them. It has been estimated that in the normal adult, the capillary bed accommodates no more than 200 to 300 ml of blood at any one time. It must be remembered that in health when arteriolar tone is normal the blood pressure can be quite low and yet capillary flow and tissue perfusion are quite adequate. (A sleeping systolic pressure of 80 mm of mercury is not uncommon.) The recording of a low blood pressure must therefore never be taken as the sole index in the diagnosis of shock.

In shock due to hypovolaemia (Fig. 7.2(b)), the activity of the sympathetic nervous system, mediated through the volume receptors of the heart and great vessels is increased. Blood levels of circulating catecholamines, adrenaline and noradrenaline are increased many-fold, reducing capillary flow by their constrictor action on arterioles. The activity of the sympathetic nervous system has different effects on different vascular beds. The kidney, skin and mesenteric flows are affected most, while there may even be an increase in myocardial flow and no change in the flow to the brain. The increased fall in pH which occurs across the capillary bed reflects the failure of the reduced capillary flow to clear the tissue metabolites (e.g. lactic acid). Catecholamines also have a direct action on the tissue cells and by interfering with intracellular enzymes are at least partly responsible for the acidosis. Even if the action of catecholamines on the microcirculation can be blocked or antagonized by the use of drugs, other harmful effects will continue while circulating blood levels remain elevated. Only when the hypovolaemia has been fully corrected will this state of affairs be reversed.

If treatment is not instituted at an early stage, tissue anoxia and accumulated metabolites relax the capillary sphincters and damage capillary endothelium. The capacity of the capillary bed may be increased three or four-fold, resulting in a loss of blood from the effective circulation by 'pooling'. Capillary permeability is increased and further fluid and plasma is lost into the tissues. These losses are added to the initial deficit and the vicious circle whereby the shocked state is perpetuated in the untreated patient, is complete. If an adequate volume of fluid is given at this stage, the vascular space is filled, the catecholamine level decreases, physiological vasodilatation occurs and capillary flow is increased.

Further delay in treatment results in sludging and aggregation of cellular blood elements which may progress to a disseminated intravascular coagulation in the capillary bed (Fig. 7.2(c)). The severe anoxia so produced will cause cell death, which may progress to organ failure. Even at this stage effective treatment (e.g. haemodyalisis for renal failure) may enable recovery to take place.

In bacteraemic shock the haemodynamic changes are not completely understood. Animal experiments suggest that shock is caused by the liberation of endotoxin from the cell wall of lysed bacteria in the blood. Endotoxin may produce the shock syndrome by a wide variety of mechanisms which may differ from bacteria to bacteria and patient to patient. Arteriovenous shunts in the microcirculation are normally closed. In bacteraemic shock however, endotoxin causes large volumes of blood to bypass the capillary beds via the shunts, possibly by a direct action on the vessel wall. Whereas in advanced hypo-volaemic shock some shunting of blood may occur, in bacteraemic shock large volumes of blood are shunted into the venous system and blood is pooled in the capacitance vessels where it is lost to the circulation. The patient becomes, in effect, hypovolaemic, sympathetic activity and catecholamine secretion are increased and the vicious circle is again complete. It has been suggested that capillary permeability is increased by a direct action on the endothelium, further exacerbating the

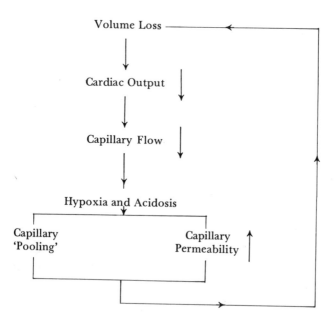

Fig. 3.7. The vicious circle in untreated shock.

hypovolaemia. Bacterial endotoxins may also increase sympathetic activity by directly stimulating the adrenal medulla and by sensitizing sympathetic receptors to the action of circulating catecholamines.

When bacteraemic shock appears to be refractory to treatment it is often due to a failure of the clinician to appreciate all the contributory factors involved. Disseminated intravascular coagulation is well described however, in certain forms of bacteraemic shock in man, and it may play a major role in some cases of refractory shock.

Blood Changes

The changes which occur in the blood in shock are extremely complex and a full description is beyond the scope of this chapter. A deficiency of coagulation factors may occur in protracted shock, possibly the result of diffuse intravascular coagulation. Blood clotting problems may also be encountered after major surgery, such as aortic aneurysm resections and open heart surgery, particularly when large volumes of stored blood have been transfused. In the shocked patient with continuing haemorrhage, when an obvious source of bleeding cannot be identified, the possibility that a coagulation defect may have arisen should always be considered.

Facilities for the estimation of serum lactate are not widely available, but when possible, the serum levels reflect the degree of acidosis in the shocked patient. Some authors have related serum lactate levels to prognosis, the higher the levels recorded, the less the chance of recovery. Special measures are seldom required however, to correct the acidosis in shock; serum lactate levels are quickly reduced once tissue perfusion is improved by therapy.

Pulmonary Changes

The lungs may be severely affected in shock, especially when due to bacteraemia. The pathological changes that have been described include atelectasis, pulmonary congestion, oedema and intra-alveolar haemorrhage. As a result of these changes there is a disturbance of ventilation-perfusion ratios in the lung.

Haemorrhage and hypotension result in pulmonary hypotension with resultant non-perfusion of ventilated alveoli. Under these conditions a proportion of the tidal volume is unable to take part in gaseous exchange due to failure of perfusion. Thus, there is an increase in the physiological dead space to tidal volume ratio which results in inadequate oxygenation of arterial blood and inadequate elimination of carbon dioxide. These changes are usually reversible providing adequate measures are taken to tide the patient over the crisis.

Cardiac Changes

In most forms of shock, the basic physiological abnormality is an inadequate cardiac output. Cardiac output is dependent upon two factors; the rate at which blood is returned to the heart and the efficiency of the cardiac pump. Myocardial cells may be inadequately perfused during severe shock and contractility is further impaired by the metabolic acidosis.

In the early stages of some forms of bacteraemic shock, when the shunting of blood through opened arterio-venous anastomoses is the predominant change, the venous return to the heart may not be reduced, and cardiac output may be normal or even increased. However, bacterial endotoxin has a direct depressant action on the myocardium and in the majority of cases, particularly the elderly, an element of cardiac failure contributes to a complicated clinical picture and must receive attention.

When treating a patient in traumatic shock due to multiple injuries, the venous return to the heart and therefore the cardiac output can be impaired by an increase in intrathoracic pressure, even after hypovolaemia has been corrected. This may be due to a tension pneumothorax, haemothorax, cardiac tamponade or intermittent positive pressure ventilation. These possibilities should always be considered when the expected recovery does not follow transfusion.

THE CLINICAL SIGNS OF SHOCK

Although modern techniques and instruments enable accurate measurement of many parameters of a patient's progress, they must not replace any aspect of a thorough examination and

clinical appraisal of a shocked patient. The clinician must be
alert to the signs and symptoms of inadequate tissue perfusion.

Whatever the mechanism whereby tissue perfusion is reduced,
the resultant fall in cardiac output and hypotension will have
maximum effect on those tissues and organs most sensitive to
anoxia, the brain and kidneys. Lowered brain perfusion will be
evident from the patient's anxiety and agitation. The patient
may well faint and may even lose consciousness on assuming
the erect posture. Poor kidney perfusion is manifest by oliguria
which may progress to anuria due to acute tubular necrosis. The
respiratory rate and volume are increased but, especially in a
slowly progressing haemorrhage, this may pass unnoticed until
syncope occurs.

In hypovolaemic shock, increased sympathetic activity is
evident from the vasoconstriction of the skin vessels leading to
pallor of the lips, hands and feet, which feel cold. Superficial
veins on the hands and feet are collapsed, capillary filling time
is increased and the patient sweats. In this stage of vasoconstriction or compensated shock a young patient may lose a considerable portion of his blood volume without any fall in blood
pressure occurring. In the elderly hypertensive patient interpretation of the patient's blood pressure at this stage is difficult and
recording a relatively high systolic pressure may give a false sense
of security. These patients however, may be in a critical state,
and any drugs which produce vasodilatation (e.g. anaesthetic
agents such as halothane) given at this stage may produce a precipitous fall in blood pressure. Similarly, a single observation of
the patient's pulse rate may be misleading, and the recording of
an increasing tachycardia should not be awaited before the
clinician's attention is drawn to the critical situation.

In normovolaemic shock tissue perfusion may be reduced
because of an abnormal vasodilatation and the shunting of blood
into venous pools. The clinical picture in bacteraemic shock
varies from patient to patient, possibly depending on the type
of bacteria responsible and also on other complicating factors
such as fluid deficiency, which commonly co-exist. In some
patients with bacteraemic shock the abnormal vasodilatation is
manifest at the onset by a warm dry skin and full peripheral
veins. These patients although appearing well on superficial
examination may be mentally confused and have a tachycardia,

211

hypotension and oliguria. In contrast to these patients, who have been described as suffering from 'warm hypotension', the remainder present with the cold, moist pallor or 'cold hypotension', common to other forms of shock. In addition to these signs a number of prodromal symptoms which may be vague and are easily missed, draw attention to the correct diagnosis. These include a complaint of chilliness, rigors, myalgia and headache. Vomiting and diarrhoea may also occur. Although the patient is not always pyrexial, a rapid rise in temperature accompanying hypotension should always suggest a bacteraemia.

If the infection in the patient with 'warm hypotension' is not controlled, the pooling of the blood and fluid shifts which occur result in what is, in effect, a hypovolaemia. Eventually the vasoconstriction in response to catecholamine secretion predominates and the patient passes into a state of 'cold hypotension'.

MONITORING THE SHOCKED PATIENT

Full assessment of the shocked patient and careful documentation of the changes which take place is the only way in which a successful outcome can be assured.

It is, of course, essential to have baseline measurements of haemoglobin, serum electrolytes and blood gases before commencing treatment and these must be repeated as frequently as the patient's condition dictates.

There are two main aims in assessing the shocked patient. First, an estimation of the fluid deficit must be made, and secondly they must provide some estimate of the ability of the pumping mechanism, that is the heart and peripheral circulation, to provide adequate tissue perfusion.

Fluid Deficit

1. *Haematocrit.* Serial measurements of the haematocrit as a guide to fluid requirements in the shocked patient, in whom pooling of blood in the peripheral circulation is occurring, can be inaccurate and misleading. Its estimation may however, be of some value especially in estimating the fluid requirements in the severely burned patient. In the patient who has bled, when fluid

deficits are complex, determination of the red blood cell mass is possibly the best index of blood requirements.

2. *Blood Volume.* Estimations which depend upon dilution of an intravenously administered radio-isotope have proved to be unreliable because the sluggish peripheral circulation in shock -prevents complete mixing of the isotope with the blood. In addition, for estimations of small deficits in blood volume to be made, it is necessary to have an accurate estimation of the patient's normal blood volume. Larger deficits in blood volume are usually apparent on clinical examination of the patient.

3. *Extracellular Fluid Volume.* An accurate and quick method of estimating ECF volume would prove invaluable in the management of the shocked patient. Unfortunately the techniques at present available again depend on dilution of a radio-isotope throughout the body fluids and interpretation of results has proved difficult. As yet, no precise bedside method is available.

4. *Central Venous Pressure* (CVP). The measurement of central venous pressure has become an invaluable aid in estimating the fluid volume requirements of the seriously ill and shocked patient. The CVP is measured in the right atrium and that part of the superior and inferior venae cavae which extends from the heart up to the first venous valves. The pressure in these veins depends on two factors: the volume of blood returning to the heart (the effective blood volume), and the efficiency of the cardiac pump. An alteration in either of these factors will tend to change the CVP. A low CVP implies a deficit in the circulating blood volume and a high CVP is due to a failing myocardium or an overloading of the circulation by an excessive administration of intravenous fluids. CVP measurement should always be used in the severely shocked patient and also whenever a patient does not respond to what is believed to be adequate fluid replacement. It is particularly helpful in the elderly patient or when cardiac failure complicates the clinical picture.

Several methods are available for introducing a central venous catheter —

(i) Puncture of the cephalic vein or one of its tributaries is often

213

the preferred method. Percutaneous puncture is usually possible, but a venous cutdown may be necessary to allow a catheter of sufficient calibre to be introduced. The catheter is gently advanced until it is manipulated into the superior vena cava, although difficulty can be experienced in negotiating the confluence of the cephalic and subclavian veins. Abduction of the arm may help at this stage. When a large catheter is introduced into a vein of small calibre the incidence of phlebitis and cellulitis in the arm is high. The same criticism applies to the use of the femoral vein for the introduction of a catheter, and for this reason the puncture of larger veins in the neck is often preferred.

(ii) The external jugular vein is usually visible and if not, it can be distended by pressure exerted with the finger at the root of the neck. It can be entered by percutaneous puncture when the patient is in the supine position with the head turned towards the opposite side. The large calibre of the jugular vein minimizes the risk of phlebitis and the only common complication of this method is a haematoma in the neck, usually when undue pressure has been used to negotiate the confluence of the external jugular and subclavian veins. If this cannot be achieved CVP recordings can be made through a shorter cannula inserted in the external jugular vein and not advanced into the superior vena cava.

(iii) The internal jugular vein may also be used by the skilled and experienced operator for introducing a catheter into the superior vena cava to provide an accurate record of the pressure in the central veins. The supine patient is positioned with the head rotated to the opposite side and the skin punctured 3 cm above the clavicle at the lateral border of the sternomastoid. An attached syringe is repeatedly aspirated to indicate when the vein is entered, as the needle is advanced towards the suprasternal notch. Alternatively, the vein may be entered by puncturing the skin between the two heads of the sternomastoid low in the neck, and advancing the needle directly backwards.

(iv) If other methods to introduce a catheter into the superior vena cava fail, the subclavian vein may be entered direct. The skin is punctured 1 cm below the midpoint of the clavicle and advanced medially at an angle of 15° to the long axis of the clavicle, aiming at the sternoclavicular joint. The vein is entered at a point beneath the medial end of the clavicle where it is related to the apical pleura medially and separated from the subclavian artery and brachial plexus behind by the insertion of the scalenus anterior. Damage to nerve, artery and lung resulting in pneumothorax and haemothorax have been recorded. This method therefore, should only be used by those experienced in the technique, when other approaches to the central veins prove unsuccessful.

The strictest aseptic precautions must be observed whenever a catheter is introduced. Failure to do so results in a large number of infected catheters from which fatal bacteraemia has been reported. The skin must be thoroughly prepared using chlorhexidine or iodine and sterile gloves should be worn by the operator.

Several varieties of plastic catheters and cannulae, specifically for recording CVP, are produced commercially. The shortest catheter which will reach the central veins should be used because the sensitivity of CVP recording and the rate at which intravenous fluids can be given through the catheter are a function of its length. In addition, damage to the myocardium has been recorded, due to the introduction of too long a catheter. When recording the pressure from the external jugular vein a short cannula (Angiocath, 14·5 cm long) is very suitable. Commercially available catheters which range in length from 20 cm to 90 cm (Intracath, E–Z cath) are available for recording via other routes. They have the advantages that they are radio-opaque, enabling their position to be checked on X-ray.

A saline manometer is the simplest and cheapest method of recording central venous pressure. Its two main disadvantages are that it does not enable a permanent continuous record to be made and that a rise in pressure fills the manometer with blood which is liable to clot. Electrical transducers are now available for continuous monitoring and recording, and are more sensitive and are easier to read than the simple manometer. The cost of these instruments however, precludes their routine use in most units. The intravenous catheter is connected through a 3-way tap to the manometer and the third limb of the tap is connected to an infusion set from which the system can be primed and rapid infusions can be given when a recording is not being taken. A fluctuation of 1 to 2 cm in the saline level with each respiration indicates that the catheter tip is correctly sited and that an accurate reading is being taken.

The actual level of CVP recorded varies widely from individual to individual and also depends upon the reference level at which the zero mark on the manometer is placed. Perhaps the most satisfactory level is a point in the mid-axillary line, approximately 10 cm from the bed, with the patient lying supine. A spirit level enables this reference point to be lined up with the zero on the manometer calibration accurately. With this as the reference level the normal range can be taken to be 5—10 cm of water. Zero to 5 cm may be considered low, 10—15 cm as high normal, and levels above 15 cm indicate a serious risk of pulmonary oedema developing. Alternatively, the sternal angle may be used as a reference point. More important than obtaining a precisely accurate initial pressure recording, is the recording of changes in the CVP which may occur during a period of observation and in response to the administration of intravenous fluids. It should be remembered that in the patient undergoing positive pressure ventilation, values 2 to 4 cm of water higher than the true CVP may be recorded.

The Efficiency of the Pumping Mechanism

1. *Heart and Blood Pressure.* It is essential that the pulse rate and blood pressure of all shocked patients are frequently and accurately recorded. Intermittent recording of the blood pressure using a sphygmomanometer may give a false low reading when the arterial pressure is less than 80 mm mercury and in the patient who does not respond rapidly to treatment, continuous monitoring of the intra-arterial pressure may be preferred. Intra-arterial pressure may be simply and accurately measured by inserting a cannula into the radial artery at the wrist and connecting it to a simple saline manometer or pressure transducer. This enables arterial pressure to be continuously observed and prompt action to be taken if any rapid deterioration occurs. An electrocardiogram monitor is invaluable for continuous observation of the heart rate and it also allows abnormal cardiac rhythms to be instantly recognized.

2. *Renal Function.* A good urine flow indicates good renal perfusion, and reflects the degree of perfusion of all other tissues. A strict record of urine output must be kept, usually necessitating catheterization of the bladder. An hourly output of less than 20 ml in the early stages of shock usually indicates inadequate tissue perfusion and the need for further therapy. In prolonged shock, when the urine output does not respond to what is considered to be adequate fluid replacement, the possibility of renal failure due to tubular necrosis should be considered. Such a patient may be given a trial with Mannitol, an osmotic diuretic, which is neither metabolized nor absorbed from the renal tubules. If the urine flow does not improve in response to a slow intravenous injection of 25 gm of Mannitol, given over a 10-minute period, then it is likely that renal damage has occurred.

Apart from its use as a diagnostic test for acute renal failure in shock, it has been suggested by experimental and clinical studies that Mannitol is effective in protecting the kidney against failure. There may, therefore, be a place for its prophylactic use from the time the patient first becomes shocked, but the increased urine output so produced must not be allowed to lull the clinician into thinking that perfusion of all the body tissues is adequate. If prescribed, its use should be limited to a maximum of 100 gm per day, for in larger doses it can induce hyponatraemia.

3. *Cardiac Output.* In the complicated clinical problem, when shock is the result of several aetiological factors such as hypovolaemia, bacteraemia and cardiac failure, accurate estimation of the cardiac output may give a valuable guide to therapy.

The indicator-dilution technique is the method most used at the present time. A bolus of the dye, indocyanine green, is injected rapidly into the venous side of the circulation, and the peak dye concentration measured in blood samples taken at a distant point (usually in arterial blood). From these estimations the cardiac output can be calculated by the application of formulae. A thermodilution method, in which a bolus of cold saline solution is injected, has recently been introduced and may prove to be a more accurate method of cardiac output estimation in the future. The results are usually expressed as the cardiac index, which relates cardiac output to the body surface area.

In the shocked patient, however, the results of cardiac output determinations may be difficult to interpret, because a normal cardiac index does not necessarily mean that tissue perfusion is satisfactory, especially when abnormal arteriovenous shunting is occurring as in bacteraemic shock. Under these circumstances repeated measurements which show that a low cardiac index is rising in response to treatment, can be a valuable guide.

MANAGEMENT AND THERAPY

The treatment of the shocked patient should be directed towards increasing tissue oxygenation by increasing the blood flow through the micro-circulation and must also aim at correcting the basic defect responsible for the shocked state. The difficult problems in treatment at the present time occur in massive trauma involving several organ systems, in bacteraemic shock, in patients in whom shock is untreated for a long time, and in patients with pre-existing conditions such as myocardial failure. Such problems are usually complex and the details of treatment will differ from patient to patient. The same general principles however, must apply to all patients and in many severely shocked patients life-saving measures will be required before there is time to make a precise diagnosis.

The patient should be nursed supine, adjusting the position to that of maximum comfort for the injured patient. In those who have recently sustained a heavy loss of blood, elevation of the legs may aid venous return to the heart whilst transfusion is commenced. The legs only should be elevated and not the whole patient positioned with the head down, because when prolonged this position is uncomfortable for the patient, may impede respiration, and may even decrease cerebral blood flow.

Obviously urgent measures must be taken to control bleeding from open wounds and to prevent continuing blood loss into the tissues around fracture sites by adequate splinting and fixation. Analgesics must be administered for the relief of pain, small repeated doses of morphia given intravenously being preferable in the severely ill patient to a large intramuscular dose, the absorption of which is uncertain when the peripheral circulation is poor.

Respiratory Function

The work of respiration may become too great for the exhausted shocked patient who may be further embarrassed by pulmonary infection, atelectasis, contusion or elevated diaphragms from abdominal distension. Evidence of early respiratory failure is most accurately provided by blood gas analysis, but it should always be remembered that in the shocked patient with adequate ventilation, the arterial oxygen saturation may be normal, and improvement in tissue oxygenation is most effectively brought about by increasing tissue perfusion.

Even when the oxygen saturation of the haemoglobin is normal, however, one can provide extra oxygen in solution in the plasma by administering a high concentration of oxygen in the inspired gases. Thus, by giving oxygen instead of room air to a shocked patient whose ventilation is adequate one can provide a significant proportion of the tissue requirements by increasing the oxygen in solution in the plasma. It is therefore always worth giving added oxygen in the presence of circulatory failure especially when there is a lowered haemoglobin. Oxygen should be administered through a nasal catheter or face mask but this route will prove inadequate for many of the complicated problems mentioned when positive pressure ventilation will be essential to survival. Certainly, if the arterial PO_2 falls below 80 mm of mercury despite added oxygen then artificial ventilation may be required. When the arterial carbon dioxide tension exceeds 45 mm of mercury, respiratory acidosis is present. When this figure reaches 60 mm of mercury assisted ventilation may need to be considered. This will necessitate endotracheal intubation or tracheostomy if rapid recovery is not expected. A cuffed tube will be necessary. The shock lung is a 'stiff' lung and considerable pressures may be required to ensure adequate ventilation.

Intravenous Fluids

When correcting a patient's fluid deficit it is necessary to assess as accurately and as quickly as possible both the volume requirement and the type of fluid which will best correct the deficit.

219

Volume Requirement. In estimating the volume of fluid required, account must first be taken of the blood losses suffered by the patient in the case of haemorrhage, which may be obvious or an occult loss into the peritoneal cavity or gut. The volume of fluid lost through fistulae or in vomiting and diarrhoea should be measured, and the electrolyte content of the loss estimated if possible. The plasma and electrolyte deficit in severely burned patients can be estimated by the application of formulae which relate the surface area burnt to fluid requirements.

In protracted shock, however, when prompt treatment has not been instituted there must be added to the above losses the blood and extracellular fluid which is lost to the effective circulation by sequestration in the capillary bed, pooling in the venous capacitance vessels and transudation through damaged capillary endothelium. Even in bacteraemic shock which occurs when the patient is in normal fluid balance, large volumes of intravenous fluids may be required to compensate for the fluid shifts and venous pooling which occurs. Not until these deficits are made good will the venous return to the heart attain normal levels and cardiac output be adequate to perfuse the tissues.

Measurement of central venous pressure gives the best practical guide to fluid volume requirements. It must always be remembered that the CVP also reflects the ability of the myocardium to cope with the additional volume infused and that in many patients a failing myocardium will require attention if adequate fluid replacement is to be accomplished. A central venous pressure of less than 2 cm of water indicates an inadequate venous return to the heart and a need for intravenous fluid therapy. It is usually preferable to administer fluids in increments of 300 ml at 15 to 20 minute intervals, rather than by a continuous infusion. This time interval allows the heart and circulation time to adapt to the additional volume and if the CVP does not rise to normal levels then further increments can be given until it does. The procedure is repeated until a normal CVP of 5 to 10 cm of water is achieved. If at this CVP the systemic arterial pressure returns to normal then the infusion can be discontinued. If the systemic pressure remains low then the infusion should be continued with great caution giving smaller increments more slowly, until the CVP rises to 14 cm. Above this level there is considerable danger of pulmonary oedema developing and throughout therapy the lungs must be frequently auscultated for the crepitations which herald its onset. Failure of the systemic pressure to rise when these high venous pressures are achieved usually indicates the necessity of treating a failing myocardium.

Type of Fluid. Military experience has shown that a marked improvement of survival figures can be brought about by the prompt and efficient treatment of traumatic and haemorrhagic shock. This is particularly relevant in the elderly where a few minutes of profound hypotension may prove fatal in a patient with coronary artery disease. In such an emergency situation volume replacement is more important than accurate replacement of the blood, electrolytes or plasma, whichever the patient may have lost. Whilst blood is being properly cross-matched for the patient whose shock is due to haemorrhage, an electrolyte solution such as Ringer Lactate may be adequate to support the circulation. If the patient's condition is very poor then an infusion of stored plasma or a colloid solution may be indicated. With continuing haemorrhage, circulatory support must be provided by the best means available while the patient is transported to the operating theatre to have, for example, a ruptured spleen removed. The types of intravenous fluids currently available and the relative merits are discussed in the following paragraphs.

(i) Blood — In the patient who has bled there is no substitute for properly cross-matched, type specified blood to make good the deficit. When prompt treatment is instituted, the patient's general condition and central venous pressure will indicate whether replacement has been adequate. If treatment is considerably delayed however, an equal volume of electrolyte solution may have to be given in addition to the shed blood volume, to compensate for the fluid shifts which occur. Under these circumstances, as in the cases where haemorrhage is accompanied by electrolyte loss, estimation of Packed Cell Volume and Red Cell Mass will give some indication of the exact volume of whole blood which is required.

If shock is profound and the need for increasing the oxygen carrying capacity of the blood is great, or if crossmatching

221

facilities are not available, the use of Rhesus negative, Group O, 'universal donor' blood with a low Anti-A titre is justified.

Blood is stored in an acid-citrate-dextrose solution and when received from the blood bank its pH is 6·6 to 7, it contains no ionized calcium, the plasma potassium is high, and it is cold. With moderate transfusions the body is able to cope with these abnormalities and provided the blood is warmed to body temperature no special measures are needed. When volumes in excess of 5 units are given rapidly however, acidosis may be increased and a deficiency of ionized calcium occurs, increasing the likelihood of cardiac arrest or ventricular fibrillation. Under these circumstances it is probably a wise precaution to give calcium gluconate or chloride (1 gramme) and sodium bicarbonate (40 milliequivalents) with each 5 units of blood.

A bleeding diathesis has been described in patients receiving massive transfusions of stored blood. Many factors may be involved, including dilutional thrombocytopaenia, fibrinolysin, disseminated intravascular coagulation and loss of the Labile Factors V and VII. The possibility that a deficiency of clotting factors may play an important role in continuing haemorrhage should always be considered and when massive transfusion is required, a transfusion of fresh blood should be given if a bleeding tendency is demonstrated. When the platelet count is adequate, fresh frozen plasma, which contains all the other clotting factors, may be given to correct the deficit.

(ii) Plasma – Pooled plasma may be used as a blood substitute in an emergency situation when waiting for whole blood to become available. It has the serious disadvantage, however, that it carries the risk of transmitting the hepatitis virus and for this reason colloid or crystalloid solutions are often preferred.

Fresh frozen plasma taken from one donor minimizes the risk of hepatitis and has the advantage that it contains all the clotting factors. It is, therefore, of considerable value in correcting the coagulation defects which may occur in the shocked patient. Fresh plasma may also be given as a means of administering protein, particularly in conditions leading to large losses of protein such as severe burns.

(iii) Colloids – The development of dextrans has provided a means of expanding the blood volume and, at the same time, maintaining a normal osmotic pressure of the blood, when whole blood is not available. Dextrans cause the transfer of fluid from the extravascular space into the blood by their osmotic action, and so they increase the circulating blood by an amount greater than their own volume. This osmotic action is related to the molecular weight of the dextran, the smaller the molecule the greater the increase in blood volume produced. The length of time the dextrans stay in the circulation is also related to the molecular weight.

Low molecular dextran (Mol. weight 40 000) has a powerful osmotic effect and may produce a shift of extracellular fluid greater in volume than the actual volume of dextran administered. For this reason, the infusion of low molecular weight dextran should always be accompanied by an electrolyte solution. It is rapidly excreted by the kidneys and its effect, therefore, only persists for a few hours.

Medium molecular dextran (Mol. weight 70 000) is excreted at a slower rate and its effect persists longer. It also has a less marked osmotic effect and is, therefore, probably the most suitable dextran to use as a blood substitute in an emergency while blood cross-match is awaited. It should be remembered that dextrans interfere with blood cross-matching and that samples for blood grouping and cross-matching should always be taken before the dextran infusion commences.

Large molecular dextran (Mol. weight 120 000) remains for a long time because it is metabolized and not excreted by the kidney. It has less osmotic effect than the lower molecular weight dextrans and therefore a larger volume must be given to produce a similar expansion of the circulating blood volume.

Dextrans are known to produce clotting defects when given in large volumes, although the exact mechanism is not fully understood. Lower molecular weight dextrans, by their osmotic action, prevent the sludging of erythrocytes and promote increased blood flow and have, therefore, been used in the treatment of ischaemic limbs. Its use in shock has recently been favoured because of this ability to lower blood viscosity and so prevent erythrocyte aggregation in low flow states. By this mechanism they may cause a bleeding tendency when given in large volumes although they are not acting as an anticoagulant as such. In addition, dextrans of large molecular size may also cause a deficit of clotting factors by promoting disseminated

223

intravascular coagulation. Their use in shock should therefore be restricted and the normal dose of 15 ml/kg body weight should not be exceeded.

(iv) Crystalloids — In recent years there has been some controversy on the value of crystalloid solutions such as Ringer's Lactate* solution, in the treatment of shock. It should be repeated that in shock due to haemorrhage, there is no substitute for correcting the deficit by the transfusion of whole blood. In an emergency situation, when blood or blood substitutes are not available, an infusion of Ringer's Lactate solution will expand the blood volume, promote blood flow and correct acidosis. This effect however, is only temporary and the lactate solution is rapidly lost from the circulation into the extracellular fluid. If the treatment has been long delayed, then the fluid shifts which occur in the microcirculation resulting in further depletion of the circulating blood volume, will require correction. This will necessitate the infusion of electrolyte solutions in addition to the transfusion of blood in volumes adequate to replace the volume shed. Estimation of the exact volume of electrolyte solution required by a patient may be difficult and the volume administered will depend on CVP and haematocrit measurements which act as a guide.

In shock due to causes other than haemorrhage, crystalloid solutions are often essential to make good the fluid deficits which complicate the clinical picture of, for example, intestinal obstruction or peritonitis. In septicaemic shock, even when occurring in patients who were previously well and in normal fluid balance, large volumes of electrolyte solutions may be required to compensate for the shunting and pooling of blood and the extracellular fluid shifts which occur.

Correction of Acidosis. Although the degree of acidosis and blood lactate levels have been related in some studies to prognosis of the shocked patient, it must be remembered that the marked acidosis which may occur reflects a severe and complex clinical situation and is not responsible per se for the high mortality. In clinical practice a persistent base deficit may have

*Ringer's Lactate: Na^+ 131 mEq/litre K^+ 5 mEq/litre
Lactate 29 mEq/litre Cl^- 111 mEq/litre
Ca^{++} 4 mEq/litre.

a pronounced effect on the blood pressure, mainly by its depressant effect on the myocardium. The increased levels of blood lactate, however, quickly return to normal once tissue perfusion is restored by adequate transfusion, even when by stored blood which is high in lactate or by lactated Ringer's solution. There is therefore, seldom a need to administer sodium bicarbonate to correct acidosis in the shocked patient. If full recovery does not follow transfusion the blood pH should be estimated and the result will indicate whether correction of acidosis is necessary. Sodium bicarbonate should never be given empirically, but only after blood pH determination, because not all shocked patients are acidotic and some may, in fact, be alkalotic, possibly due to hyperpnoea.

Septicaemic Shock. To overcome the infection two principles must be remembered. First, the patient must be treated with an adequate dose of the antibiotic to which the organism is sensitive, and second, the source of the infection must be eliminated. In addition to the measures taken to overcome the infection, full attention must, of course, be paid to correcting the fluid deficits which may pre-exist and which will occur in the established septicaemic shock. Saline or Ringer's Lactate Solution are probably the best fluids to use, the volume being controlled by CVP measurement as previously described. Blood cultures should be taken, and also cultures from all possible sources of infection, such as wounds and urine, before anti-bacterial therapy is started.

Antibiotics. The clinician may have a good idea as to the likely pathogen from a knowledge of pre-existing sources of infection, such as the urinary tract or major gastro-intestinal surgery. Previous cultures of urine, peritoneal pus, infected bile or burns will point to the infecting organism and to the most appropriate antibiotic. The physician's knowledge of recent infections which have occurred in the unit in which the patient is nursed may also be a valuable guide. In the majority of cases however, no such knowledge is available and it is necessary to commence treatment with a broad spectrum antibiotic or combination of antibiotics. Certainly in such a potentially serious condition it is never justified to await the results of cultures before commencing treatment. *Kanamycin Sulphate* (10–15 mg per kg body weight per day in three or four divided doses, up to a maximum of 1 g per day) may be used when a gram negative infection due to Escherichia coli or proteus species is suspected. The dose should be modified for age and renal function and it should probably only be used in hospitals where the facility for estimating blood levels exists. *Gentamycin* (3–5 mg per kg body weight per day in three divided doses) may be used in similar circumstances and has the added advantage of being active against Pseudomonas Pyocyanae and Staphylococcus aureus. Both Kanamycin and Gentamycin are ototoxic drugs and should be used with caution when the urinary output is less than 30 ml per hour. *Cephalothin* is a broad spectrum antibiotic which is free from the above side effects, and is active against gram negative and positive organisms with the exception of Pseudomonas Pyocanae. This is now often preferred as the antibiotic of choice in cases where no bacteriological information is available. It may be given intramuscularly, but the intravenous route enables higher blood levels to be obtained quicker and more certainly (150 mg per kg body weight in divided doses). Cephalothin should be preferred to Cephaloridine which may cause renal damage in high doses, especially in patients who may already have some impairment of renal function. Combinations of antibiotics may be given to critically ill patients when the organism is unknown, to produce an additive effect or possibly a synergistic action. If the bacteraemia is known to be due to Pseudomonas, then Carbenicillin sodium (300 mg per kg body weight per day by divided doses) may be given in addition to Gentamycin. Both antibiotics should be given separately by bolus injections every six hours. For other severe infections combinations of Cephalothin with Methicillin, Kanamycin or Gentamycin have all been recommended. When a mixed bacterial infection, which includes gram negative anaerobes is suspected the above antibiotics may not be effective and Clindamycin (20 mg per kg per day orally) or its parenteral counterpart Lincomycin hydrochloride may be prescribed in combination with another antibiotic.

Steroids. There has been considerable debate on the value of corticosteroids in shock. This arose from the original belief that

adrenal insufficiency contributed to the shock syndrome and
the doses of steroids which were first prescribed were those
which were considered adequate to replace this deficiency. It
has now been shown however, that circulating levels of hydrocortisone are increased and not decreased in shock. In cardiac
and hypovolaemic shock the levels attained appear to be
adequate and no convincing evidence has been provided to show
that the administration of corticosteroids, even when given in
very large pharmacological doses, is of any benefit. In septicaemic shock however, experimental and clinical observation
has shown that massive doses of steroids which produce blood
levels far in excess of the normal physiological response, are
beneficial. The mode of action of pharmacological doses of
steroids is not clear, but it is evident that the beneficial effect is
due to several modes of action. They appear to have an
inotropic action on the heart improving the function of the
failing myocardium in septicaemia and also a vasodilating
action on the peripheral circulation, which improves tissue
perfusion. In addition large doses of steroids also have a stabiliz-
ing effect on cells, preventing the propagation of tissue injury
by released proteases. It is now accepted that hydrocortisone in
a dose of 50 mg/kg/day, given in divided doses at six-hourly
intervals is beneficial in septicaemic shock. Fluid deficits must
be made good before steroid therapy is commenced because
hypotension from vasodilatation might otherwise result. Steroid
therapy need only be continued for 36–48 hours when they
may be stopped abruptly if recovery has occurred.

Surgery. When fluid replacement, antibiotic and steroid
therapy have led to an improvement in the patient's general
condition, the appropriate steps must be taken to treat any
underlying surgical abnormalities. Full recovery will not take
place until the source of the bacteraemia has been dealt with.
Septicaemia due to cholangitis, for example, is likely to
continue until any obstruction of the bile duct is relieved and
the infected bile adequately drained. The condition of a patient
with acute fulminating ulcerative colitis may in part be due to
septicaemia, and will not improve until colectomy is performed.
This may mean subjecting a patient who is desperately ill to an
operation but it is often essential before recovery can take
place.

Vasoactive Drugs

Vasoconstrictors. In the past sympathomimetic drugs have been used in the treatment of shock. An infusion of noradrenaline given to the shocked patient may comfort the physician by producing a rise in blood pressure but this is brought about by arteriolar constriction which has the effect of further reducing tissue perfusion and oxygenation. Soon after commencing the infusion, the venous return to the heart may increase because the peripheral veins also contract, but this is only a temporary phenomenon and subsequently venous return and cardiac output fall. The use of sympathomimetic agents in shock therefore, usually marks the beginning of a downward progression towards death, for they worsen the basic physiological defect of lowered tissue perfusion. They probably have no place in the modern therapy of the shocked patient.

Vasodilators. In recent years attention has been directed to more drugs which block the action of adrenaline on the micro-circulation. It has been suggested that there are two types of adrenergic receptors; alpha and beta receptors. The alpha effects are largely excitatory except for intestinal relaxation, and by acting at these receptors circulating catecholamines in shock are responsible for vasoconstriction. The beta effects are thought to be inhibitory except for myocardial stimulation. Drugs which block the alpha effects of adrenaline have been recommended in the treatment of refractory shock on the grounds that they increase tissue perfusion by relaxation of arterioles. This group of drugs include phenoxybenzamine (Dibenzyline), phentolamine (Rogitine) and chlorpromazine (Largactil).

Phenoxybenzamine. This is the most widely recommended drug in the treatment of the shocked patient. A dose of 1 mg per kg body weight, diluted in 500 ml of dextrose or saline, is given by slow intravenous infusion over a period of not less than one hour. It must be remembered that its full effects may not be seen for one hour after administration and that they persist for 24 hours. Great caution must be observed in administering this drug. Phenoxybenzamine, by arteriolar and venular relaxation, may produce a large increase in the vascular capacitance, resulting in a marked fall in blood pressure. It should never be given

228

unless recovery has not occurred with full replacement of any fluid deficit under CVP control. Whilst phenoxybenzamine is being given, further fluid therapy, often amounting to several litres, may be required to compensate for the vasodilatation.

The use of phenoxybenzamine in shock would be confined to those patients whose condition does not improve after instituting the other measures outlined in treatment. The major stimulus to catecholamine secretion in shock is hypovolaemia and adequate fluid replacement will reduce circulating levels, breaking the vicious circle and leading to recovery in the majority of patients. In septicaemia however, even when the circulating volume is adequate, catecholamines continue to circulate, possibly due to direct stimulation of the adrenal medulla by bacterial endotoxins. Under these circumstances massive doses of corticosteroids may prove effective, in part, due to their vasodilating action, but if not phenoxybenzamine should be considered. Patients in whom the picture is further complicated by myocardial insufficiency may also benefit from the reduction in the pressure work load on the heart, produced by the vasodilatation.

Phentolamine. This drug may also be used for its alpha-blocking effect, but its action is short and it must be given by continuous intravenous infusion.

Chlorpromazine. The moderate alpha-blocking action of chlorpromazine has led to it being recommended in the treatment of shock. However, in doses which are effective it also has a significant depressant action on the central nervous system, an action which is not always desirable in the shocked patient.

Cardiac Glycosides

Cardiac failure may necessitate therapy with digitalis or other antiarrhythmic therapy. This aspect of treatment must not be neglected, especially in the elderly. Progressive cardiac failure may be an important factor in refractory shock and it has been recommended that all shocked patients over the age of 50 years should be digitalized. After fluid replacement, if the CVP remains high in the face of hypotension, then treatment of cardiac failure should be commenced. The rapidly acting cardiac glycoside ouabain is probably most suitable because it is rapidly effective and more quickly eliminated from the body than the other glycosides.

Isoprenaline (Isoproterenol, Isuprel) acts by stimulation of betareceptors to produce vasodilatation in the microcirculation of voluntary muscles and an increase in the rate and force of myocardial contraction. It has, therefore, been advocated in the treatment of septicaemic shock. Most shocked patients, however, have a tachycardia, and when this is marked isoprenaline is unlikely to produce any significant increase in cardiac output. In addition, its use when not carefully controlled, may precipitate dangerous cardiac arrhythmias. Isoprenaline may occasionally be of value in the already digitalized patient and should always be used under strict ECG control. It is given, diluted by saline, by continuous intravenous infusion, in a dose of 3 to 15 microgrammes per minute.

REFRACTORY SHOCK

Patients who do not respond to the initial treatment which is instituted are often considered to have passed into a state of 'refractory shock', a term which implies that recovery is unlikely. In the majority of cases this is due to a failure on the part of the clinician to recognize a major contributing factor. With thorough and careful patient monitoring such problems should rarely be encountered, but when faced with refractory shock the following possibilities should always be borne in mind:

1. Continuing blood loss.
2. Inadequate fluid replacement.
3. Cardiac tamponade. Pneumothorax.

In a patient suffering from multiple injuries which include the chest, the chest radiograph taken on admission to hospital may be within normal limits. If the patient fails to respond to the initial treatment, the possibility that a haemopericardium or tension pneumothorax may have developed should always be considered, and a repeat radiograph ordered.

Shock

    4. Concomitant bacteraemic shock.
        The possibility that infection may be playing a signifi-
cant role is often not recognized, or treatment of a known
infection may be inadequate.
    5. Myocardial insufficiency.

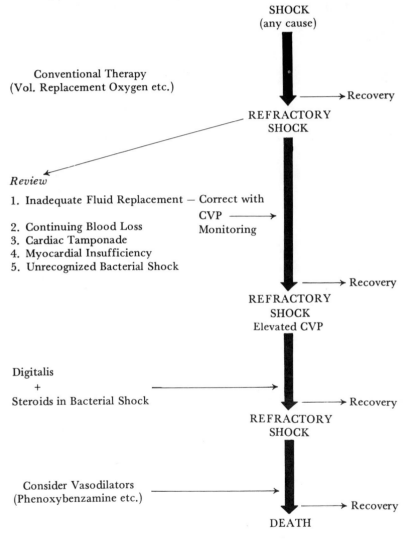

Fig. 7.4. Outline for treatment of shock.

231

The broad outline for the treatment of the shocked patient is summarized in Fig. 7.4. Since no two clinical situations are identical and in any individual patient the clinical picture can change rapidly, no fixed outline of management can be recommended. An awareness on the part of the clinician of all possible factors involved, careful patient monitoring and prompt institution of the correct therapy, will inevitably lead to increased survival in shock.

FURTHER READING

Weil, M. H. and Shubin, H. (1967). *Diagnosis and Treatment of Shock.* Williams and Wilkins.

Hardaway, R. M. (1965). Microcoagulation in shock, *Amer. J. Surg.,* 110, 298.

Hardaway, R. M. *et al.* (1967). Intensive study and treatment of shock in man, *J. Amer. Med. Ass.,* 199, 115.

Irving, M. H. (1968). The sympatho-adrenal factor in haemorrhagic shock, *Ann. Roy. Coll. Surg.,* 42, 367.

Hershey, S. G. *et al.* (1971). *Septic Shock in Man,* Churchill/Livingstone.

Chapter 8

The Intensive Therapy of Acute Poisoning

P. MARSDEN

INTRODUCTION

DIAGNOSIS

INITIAL ASSESSMENT

BASIC PRINCIPLES OF INTENSIVE THERAPY IN ACUTE POISONING

POISONING BY PARTICULAR AGENTS

INTRODUCTION

Acute poisoning is now a major medical issue. Cases of poisoning make up over 10 per cent of all emergency medical admissions in some areas and the overall total mortality from poisoning continues to rise. An understanding of the basic principles of management of the poisoned patient is therefore essential if treatment is to be methodical and the results improved. This chapter is concerned primarily with medical management of the poisoned patient but it must never be forgotten that the whole patient problem may be wider than this. Most cases of poisoning are self-induced, either with true suicidal intent or, in the vast majority of cases, as a manipulative gesture. Accidental poisoning is rare except in children. There is unfortunately no clear

233

relationship between the severity of the medical problem in an acutely poisoned patient and any underlying social or psychiatric problem that may exist and it is therefore advisable always to obtain a psychiatric opinion after the patient has recovered. An extremely useful development in recent years to aid the diagnosis and management of acute poisoning in this country is the establishment of The National Poisons Information Service. These centres provide round the clock advice at the minimal inconvenience of a telephone call. A list of the centres is included at the end of the chapter.

DIAGNOSIS

This is not always easy. Most cases of poisoning have an altered state of consciousness and the patient's history may be difficult to obtain. It is essential to make use of all sources of information by questioning relatives, ambulance drivers or policemen as to the circumstances of the case, or the condition of the patient in the previous days or weeks. Details of the patient's past medical or social history may have enormous relevance to early diagnosis and management and should be obtained as soon as possible. A telephone call to the general practitioner or local dispensing pharmacist may solve problems of drug prescription or identification, and tablets and capsules must always be kept safely and not mislaid.

The evidence for poisoning should always be reviewed and if the diagnosis is presumptive, this should be stated. Unconscious patients are a source of special concern in this respect and careful examination of the nervous system is mandatory. Where abnormal or lateralizing neurological signs are found, the diagnosis of poisoning must be considered most carefully and organic neurological disease excluded as far as possible.

INITIAL ASSESSMENT OF THE PROBLEM

Speed is essential, so that the problems can be defined and effective therapy commenced. The doctor who is first faced with a case of alleged poisoning must as well as obtaining available history, examine the patient quickly in order to grade approximately his functional state, and confirm the diagnosis.

Conscious level should be assessed. A clinically useful grading is:

1. Conscious and alert.
2. Drowsy but responsive to verbal command.
3. Unconscious but responsive to minimal painful stimuli.
4. Unconscious and responsive only to maximum painful stimuli.
5. Unconscious and unresponsive to pain.

The grades are numbered for convenience. It is more important to detail the actual conscious level found than to define it by a number, as this may be uninterpretable or worse, wrongly interpreted by another person. Later neurological examination must be complete including documentation of neck stiffness and state of the fundi and tympanic membranes. Respiratory function should be assessed. Respiratory rate, the presence of under or over ventilation should be noted and if possible minute volumes of respiration recorded with a spirometer. Presence or absence of cyanosis is noted, and the chest briefly examined. The purpose of the assessment is to decide if ventilatory function is adequate or if urgent measures are required. These may take the form of insertion of a pharyngeal airway, or endotracheal tube, removal of foreign bodies from the pharynx, aspiration of vomitus occluding the airways, or immediate initiation of artificial ventilation. In general a minute volume of less than 4 litres is inadequate and blood gas estimation may confirm respiratory failure.

The circulatory status of the patient should be similarly assessed with recordings of pulse and blood pressure and any evidence of shock, cardiac failure or dysrhythmia noted. The patient's temperature should be recorded if necessary with a low reading thermometer (which should always be available) and note made of the state of hydration including the passage of urine.

The doctor should now be in a position to decide if the diagnosis of poisoning is likely and if so, whether it is minimal or if real depression of systemic function is likely to supervene. In general, the patient should be admitted to hospital however mild the medical problem as there may be an undefined large psychiatric problem but if serious depression of function exists in any system the patient should ideally be cared for in an intensive therapy unit.

BASIC PRINCIPLES OF INTENSIVE THERAPY IN ACUTE POISONING

The basic principles of treatment of a case of poisoning may be considered as follows:

1. Identification.
2. Removal.
3. Prevention of further absorption.
4. Use of antidotes.
5. Modification of the body's handling of the poison by excretion or metabolism.
6. Support of vital functions and maintenance of normal physiology.
7. Symptomatic relief.

Identification

The identification of tablets, capsules or domestic substances is important but in practice should not be allowed to take up too much time at first. Blood or urine samples should always be taken however for analysis later or forensic use. Telephone calls to the general practitioner or pharmacist may help. Samples of poisons should always be saved.

Removal of Poison

When a patient has ingested poison it may be possible to prevent further absorption from the gastrointestinal tract. In the past, vomiting has been induced with emetic drugs such as apomorphine for this purpose. This is dangerous as the effects are unpredictable, and they should in general not be used. Even the induction of vomiting by the mechanical stimulation of the pharynx may carry the danger of inhalation of vomitus in the drowsy patient.

Gastric aspiration and lavage is widely practised though firm evidence for its value is sparse. In general the procedure is likely to produce a worthwhile recovery of drug only when it is performed within three hours of ingestion and this can be adopted as a rule of thumb. Acute salicylate poisoning is the exception as aspirin tablets may be recovered from the stomach for a long time after ingestion, and gastric aspiration and lavage is worth undertaking at any stage in cases of aspirin poisoning.

Having decided to wash out the stomach, attention must be given to the patient's reflex function. If protective coughing and gagging reflexes are in any way impaired it is safer to insert a cuffed endotracheal tube before commencing in order to protect the lungs against aspiration.

A wide bore tube should be introduced, with the patient positioned head down and on the left side. The stomach is aspirated and then lavage carried out with 200 ml aliquots of tap water. The stomach should be aspirated dry at the end of the procedure, which is usually reached when it is evident that further drug is not being removed.

Prevention of Further Absorption

Acidic and alkaline substances can be neutralized preventing further effect. Adsorbants such as activated charcoal may occasionally be useful. The absorption of iron from the gastro-intestinal tract can be prevented by oral doses of desferri-oxamine but the applications of this type of treatment are few otherwise.

Antidotes

Specific antidotes exist for very few poisons. Even substances such as nalorphine in morphine poisoning are not complete anti-dotes. Other examples are atropine and PAM in anticholinester-ase poisoning and chelating agents, dimercaprol, EDTA, penicillamine and desferrioxamine. Some 'antidotes' are no longer used. Analeptic agents such as bemegride or nikethamide have no part to play in the routine management of poisoning by centrally depressant drugs. Bemegride is not a specific barbi-turate antagonist and its use is attended by violent fluctuations in conscious level and sometimes convulsions.

MODIFICATION OF EXCRETION OR METABOLISM

Forced Diuresis Regimes

The rationale of such regimes lies in increasing the renal excretion of a poison. It follows that the method will be more successful for drugs which are predominantly excreted by the kidney under normal circumstances, and can not be expected to help much where this is not the case. A second concept in induced diuresis regimes is that invoked by changing the pH of the infusion, to provide an alkaline or on occasions an acidic diuresis.

Forced diuresis regimes involve the infusion of large volumes of fluid intravenously in a short period of time and should not be started in patients who show clinical evidence of cardio-vascular disease. A history of angina, the presence of cardiac failure or pulmonary oedema from any cause would contra-indicate the regime. Similarly, a history of renal failure should alert the physician. The blood urea and electrolytes should be known before a forced diuresis regime is started and periodic estimations throughout treatment are essential. In addition it is wise to estimate arterial blood gases and urinary SG or osmolality.

The second concept is based on the physiology of the renal excretion of weak acids and bases, and is best illustrated by example.

Aspirin (acetyl salicylic acid) is a weak acid and dissociated in alkaline solutions. The dissociated radical acetylsalicylate is not fat soluble and is reabsorbed less readily by the renal tubular epithelium. It follows that if the urine is rendered alkaline, re-absorption of salicylate will be less and hence renal excretion will be greater. The same principle but in reverse applies to substances such as quinine, chloroquine or amphetamine which are best excreted in an acidic urine.

Methods

Forced Alkaline Diuresis. The patient is put on to an hourly fluid balance chart and the bladder is catheterized. Fluid is given intravenously as follows:

238

1. Sodium bicarbonate 1·2%   500 ml
2. 5% Dextrose   500 ml
3. 5% Dextrose in N/5 saline   500 ml

These infusion fluids should be given in this order to a total infusion volume of 2 litres in the first hour and 1 litre in each subsequent hour. The patient may be dehydrated initially and it may be necessary to give fluid at the rate of 2 litre per hour until an adequate diuresis is established. Potassium salts should not be added to the infusion fluid until the patient has passed at least 1 litre of urine and then should be given as KCl 1 g to every alternate 500 ml bottle. This infusion rate may have to be increased if the serum potassium falls. The pH of the urine should be measured with universal indicator and if below 7, more $NaHCO_3$ should be given. Careful and repeated clinical examinations of jugular venous pressure, respiratory rate and lung bases is necessary. Should the hourly fluid balance exceed 1·5 litres positive balance, an injection of frusemide 40 mg should be given intravenously and the infusion rate slowed. If the patient is unresponsive to pain or in the presence of hypotension or shock, a central venous pressure line should be inserted. Calcium gluconate 10 ml of 10% solution should be given if the serum calcium falls. The regime should be continued until the patient is clearly recovering consciousness or the serum salicylate level is in the therapeutic range if the case is salicylate poisoning.

Forced Acid Diuresis. It is sometimes necessary in severe cases of quinine, chloroquine or amphetamine overdosage to use this regime.

1. 5% Dextrose + 1·5 g ammonium chloride   500 ml
2. 5% Dextrose   500 ml
3. 5% Dextrose N/5 saline   500 ml

Fluid should be given in the above order at an initial rate of 1 litre per hour and then at 500 ml per hour. Otherwise the regime is as for forced alkaline diuresis except that it is essential to monitor the serum electrolytes and pH closely. Hourly specimens of urine should be tested for pH.

Dialysis Regimes. Peritoneal dialysis and haemodialysis may both be employed in the management of acute poisoning by substances that are dialysable through either the partially selective peritoneal membrane or the membranes used in the artificial kidney.* For details of the techniques, see chapter on Renal Failure.

Supportive Therapy

The support of vital functions and symptomatic relief constitute the mainstay of treatment in most cases of poisoning. This is not a negative concept but a valuable and positive therapeutic regime which has for instance been most responsible in reducing the mortality from acute barbiturate poisoning from 25% in 1945 to the present low figures of 1−2%.

Intensive Nursing Care

This is of the utmost importance. A high standard of nursing care is essential to the success of the supportive regime.

The patient should be turned hourly to relieve pressure on weight bearing areas of skin. Passive limb movements and attention to limb posture are equally important to avoid later complications of stiff muscles and joints and compression lesions of peripheral nerves. Skin care should be thorough with regular bathing and application of protective dressings to excoriated areas. Bullous lesions should be treated as superficial ulcers and any infection dealt with promptly.

Respiratory toilet is of the utmost importance. Dentures should be removed and the pharynx kept moist. Regular hourly suction of the pharynx and endotracheal tube if in situ help to prevent the accumulation of secretions and may be coupled with percussion of the chest.

One of the nurse's main tasks is the regular and thorough observation of the patient. Blood pressure, pulse, central venous pressure, respiration, conscious level, fluid input and urinary output and the calculation of fluid balance must all be recorded at half-hourly intervals. In many cases continuous monitoring of the ECG is necessary and the whole adds up to a heavy burden on nursing staff. In such circumstances, maintenance of morale

*Because of the relative inefficiency of peritoneal dialysis, it is rarely of significant value for the removal of poisons.

and a sense of identity between the various medical and paramedical disciplines contributes greatly to the success of the unit and to patient care within it.

Fluid and Electrolyte Balance. Many unconscious patients have lain for a considerable period of time with inadequate fluid intake and dehydration is therefore common. It is advisable to correct the fluid and electrolyte deficits by intravenous infusion. Provided no special situation such as vomiting or hyperpyrexia exists and there is no obvious electrolyte balance, it is in general sufficient to give dextrose saline (5% dextrose in N/5 N saline) in quantities to correct any initial deficit (usually 1–2 litres over six to eight hours) and then continue the infusion to provide adequate urine volumes of 1–2 litres per day. Blood urea and electrolytes should be estimated at least daily and potassium chloride added to the infusion fluid to maintain a normal serum potassium. In no case should potassium salts be given intravenously before the patient has passed at least 1 litre of urine, and the infusion rate should never exceed 1 g of potassium chloride per hour.

Bladder Catheterization. This is indicated where a patient is in acute retention of urine with or without incontinence or to differentiate between anuria and retention of urine. Catheterization is also usually required as part of a forced diuresis regime where it is essential to have accurate hourly fluid balance data. It must not be done routinely in the unconscious patient. Whenever a urinary catheter is inserted, full aseptic technique must be employed. Regular urine specimens must be sent for bacterial culture while it is *in situ* and a mid-stream urine specimen should be sent for examination after the catheter has been removed.

Antibiotics

Prophylactic antibiotics are contraindicated, but should be used promptly to treat actual infections of the respiratory or urinary tracts or elsewhere. Sufficient evidence of infection may be clinical or radiological rather than bacteriological, and it is important not to delay adequate therapy for an early broncho-pneumonia because bacteriological proof may not yet be available.

Physiotherapy

Passive limb movements and simple chest percussion are part of the routine care of the unconscious patient but must be supplemented by more intensive physiotherapy where broncho-pneumonia has set in, or aspiration of secretions resulted in lobar collapse. In some cases bronchoscopy may be required.

General Care

While the patient is in the Intensive Therapy Unit he will be assessed in detail at least twice daily by medical staff. Frequent re-examination of the patient, careful attention to routine observations and the functional state of the major systems all contribute to the supportive regime. Adequate radiological and pathological services must be available. A chest X-ray is essential in any patient who has been unconscious to exclude occult collapse of a lobe and in some acutely ill patients on mechanical ventilation, daily X-rays may be needed. Similarly frequent estimations of blood urea and electrolytes, blood gases, and other tests are needed and together with haematological and bacteriological requests make adequate pathological services a major factor in contributing to the success of the unit.

Special Procedures

In addition to the more general types of supportive therapy described above, special measures may be used to support the function of a failing system and correct obvious abnormalities. Special measures to treat hypotension, shock or cardiac dysrhythmias may be required. Renal failure may need dialysis, acute cerebral oedema may respond to mannitol infusion or steroid therapy and fits to anticonvulsants.

Mechanical ventilation should be used where respiratory function is inadequate. In general, a minute volume of less than 4 litres can be considered inadequate and blood gases should be estimated. Further discussion of the indications for mechanical ventilation can be found in the chapter on respiratory failure.

POISONING BY PARTICULAR AGENTS

List of contents in alphabetical order with page numbers

BARBITURATES

Acute barbiturate poisoning is still the commonest single cause of poisoning in this country. It therefore constitutes a major medical and social problem.

The frequency with which barbiturate drugs are prescribed no doubt contributes greatly to the incidence of poisoning by overdosage. The number of proprietary preparations is enormous and many, like 'Tuinal', contain mixtures of different barbiturates. The classical short and medium acting barbiturates such as pentobarbitone (Nembutal) and amylobarbitone (Amytal) respectively are in much greater clinical usage than longer acting preparations such as phenobarbitone (Luminal) or barbitone (Veronal) and hence poisoning with them is much commoner.

Presentation

The barbiturates are depressant drugs. On the central nervous system overdosage primarily results in impaired conscious level which may be profound. Accurate grading of the level of unconsciousness as specified earlier helps to give a reliable index of the severity of the case when seen and repeated observations of the conscious level are the best index of the course of the illness.

Muscle tone is reduced in barbiturate overdosage, the limbs being flaccid and the reflexes generally depressed. Plantar responses are flexor unless there is anoxic brain damage. The pupils are equal and the pupillary reflexes to light are maintained. The eyes retain the power of conjugate movement. Unfortunately the size of the pupils, the depression of limb reflexes and the retention or loss of the corneal reflex are all too variable to give a reliable guide to the severity of the case which is best judged from the conscious level. Lateralizing signs in the nervous system or pyramidal signs are in general not features of barbiturate overdosage and their presence should alert the doctor to other possible causes. Fits may however occur as a withdrawal phenomenon.

A depressant effect is also seen in the effects of cardiovascular and respiratory function. A central action in reducing vasometer tone and a direct toxic action on the musculature of the peripheral vessels and myocardium both contribute to produce bradycardia and hypotension. Low venous tone produces pooling of blood in the limbs with cold extremities, peripheral cyanosis and oedema. Direct depression of the central control of respiration leads to hypoventilation with consequent respiratory failure, and involvement of hypothalamic centres to the characteristic hypothermia.

The classical picture then of severe barbiturate poisoning is of a deeply unconscious patient with slow pulse, low blood pressure and depressed respiration. The temperature is often subnormal and the limbs flaccid with depressed reflexes but no lateralizing signs. Severe cases unresponsive to pain may also develop a degree of paralytic ileus and acute renal failure may occur following hypotension.

Treatment. The mainstay of treatment of acute barbiturate poisoning is supportive therapy. As mentioned earlier it was the abandonment of the use of stimulant drugs such as bemegride and the introduction of supportive regimes which has led to the enormous reduction in mortality from this condition in the last twenty-five years.

After the initial assessment of the patient and transfer to the intensive therapy unit, the nursing and observational regimes outlined are started. If the body temperature is low, active heating is avoided unless the temperature is below 30°C when it constitutes a serious danger to life. In these circumstances, steroids should be given as hydrocortisone 100 mg i.v. 6-hourly and the patient covered with blankets. Hypotension may give rise to anxiety but provided the patient continues to pass urine there is no real danger. Should the systolic blood pressure fall below 70 mm Hg, the first active measure is to elevate the legs. This reduces the peripheral pooling of blood, increases the cardiac output and is often all that is required. It should be noted that respiratory insufficiency may itself produce hypotension and so it is wise to review the adequacy of ventilatory function whenever hypotension occurs. If these measures do not produce a satisfactory response, then pressor agents may be given. Metaraminol bitartrate (Aramine) is satisfactory in a dose of 5 mg intramuscularly. It should not be given intravenously as there is a danger of cardiac arrhythmias or myocardial infarction. The use of pressor agents would seem logical in view of the peripheral vasodilation but as renal arteriolar constriction may occur, they should be used with caution. The smallest dose effective in raising the systolic blood pressure to a safe level (85—100 mm Hg) should be used and repeated at intervals determined by the clinical response. In general it is rare for repeated injections to be necessary. If clinical shock supervenes the above measures may be sufficient but it may be necessary to give plasma expanders such as dextran as the circulating blood volume is low in barbiturate overdosage. In such circumstances a central venous pressure line should be inserted and fluid given to maintain this at normal values. Blood gases should be estimated and hypoxaemia or acidosis corrected appropriately. Hydrocortisone in a dose of 100 mg 6-hourly may be of value.

The main cause for concern with the blood pressure level is the possibility of renal damage. If the patient becomes oliguric, it is first necessary to exclude pre-renal causes. Examination of any urine available for casts, SG and albumin and estimation of urinary urea and sodium concentrations may help to decide this but it is essential to correct any hypovolaemia by infusion of fluid until the central venous pressure is normal and the use of an osmotic diuretic such as 200 ml of 10% mannitol may cause the patient to pass urine.

If oliguria is on the basis of acute tubular necrosis and the patient is still unconscious, haemodialysis is the treatment of choice. If the patient has recovered from the acute effects of the drug, the renal failure should be managed routinely.

Careful observation of respiratory function is essential, preferably with the use of a spirometer. All cases of acute barbiturate poisoning should receive oxygen therapy by mask or nasal spectacles, unless there is significant hypercapnia. Blood gases should be estimated if the minute volume drops below 4 litres. Artificial ventilation should be commenced whenever the indications outlined in the Respiratory Failure chapter are fulfilled.

The position of treatment by forced alkaline diuresis must be considered. In recent years a vogue to use this treatment in acute barbiturate poisoning has existed, but except in the case of the long acting barbiturates, the benefit is probably extremely slight. Barbitone is 100% renally excreted and phenobarbitone 25% but shorter acting drugs are largely metabolized in the liver, are more protein bound and are less ionized at urine pH values achieved by forced alkaline diuresis. As most cases of barbiturate overdosage encountered clinically are with the short and medium acting drugs, it follows that this method of treatment is rarely justified in barbiturate poisoning. The place of haemodialysis likewise has probably been overestimated. Most cases of barbiturate over-dosage will recover on supportive therapy alone and haemo-dialysis should be reserved for those patients who are deeply comatose and unresponsive to painful stimuli who fail to improve, or deteriorate after 24–48 hours on a full supportive regime. The value of estimating the level of barbiturate in the blood as a guide to prognosis or treatment has also probably been overestimated. Levels of 3 mg % for short acting drugs and 10 mg % for long acting drugs have been taken as indications for dialysis but there is no fixed relationship between the blood level and how the patient will respond excepting that failure of high blood barbiturate levels to fall during supportive therapy may be a guide to the need for haemodialysis. The assessment of the patient's condition must be an essentially clinical one but it is however of the utmost importance that samples of blood and urine are taken and saved for possible forensic use.

SALICYLATE POISONING

Acute salicylate poisoning usually results from taking aspirin tablets. Aspirin is the most commonly taken analgesic and is included in numerous proprietary products. Furthermore, it is available without prescription. The incidence of salicylate poisoning is 12–13% of all poisonings and is rising and though this is not as common as barbiturate poisoning, the mortality is greater particularly in children.

Presentation and Biochemistry

The patient is usually restless, alert and orientated. Drowsiness or coma is unusual in salicylate poisoning but this must be appreciated and the doctor must not assume from the fact that the patient is fully conscious that the case is not serious. Depression of consciousness is more common in children where it is a grave sign indicating metabolic acidosis.

Tinnitus and deafness are common and hyperventilation follows a direct action of the drug on the central control of respiration. Excess sweating and elevation of body temperature lead to dehydration. Vomiting is also common and fluid loss may lead·to shock. Acute renal failure occurs following shock and a direct toxic action of salicylate on the renal tubules.

Aspirin also causes gastric haemorrhage from a direct mucosal action and hypoprothrombinaemia may occur to increase the risk of haematemesis. Hyper and hypoglycaemia may both occur.

The more serious feature of salicylate poisoning and certainly mortality from respiratory or cardiac arrest are consequent upon the disturbance of acid-base equilibrium that occurs. This is a mixture of metabolic acidosis resulting from increased metabolic rate and the presence of salicylic acid in the blood, and a respiratory alkalosis that results from the secondary stimulation of respiration by salicylate. Respiratory alkalosis is usually accompanied by hypokalaemia. There is a difference in response of adults and children to acute salicylate poisoning in that children tend to pass on to the more dangerous state of acidosis more quickly than adults who maintain their blood pH at or above normal.

Diagnosis. Hyperpyrexia and hyperventilation may lead to an initial diagnosis of pneumonia where no history is available and the finding of a shocked, restless and sweating patient to a suspicion of septicaemia, or even hypoglycaemia which itself can occur as a consequence of salicylate overdosage, due to increased peripheral utilization of glucose. The more usual diagnostic difficulty is that confusion with diabetic keto-acidosis may occur. Salicylates in large dosage can precipitate hyperglycaemia; ketosis occurs in both conditions, in addition to which both salicylates and ketones give a positive ferric chloride reaction in the urine. Differentiation is by pre-boiling which removes ketones. The distinction is made on the history, discrepancy between the blood sugar level and the clinical state of the patient and of course actual estimation of salicylate when poisoning is suspected.

Treatment. It cannot be too strongly emphasized that acute salicylate poisoning is a dangerous condition with an appreciable mortality (over 200 deaths per year in England and Wales). Furthermore the assessment of the severity of an individual case is difficult. There is little correlation between symptoms and signs of salicylism and mortality and the fact that the patient is conscious may lull the inexperienced doctor into a sense of false security concerning the urgency of the case. The best-guide to severity is the blood salicylate level but even here there are pitfalls. Note should be taken if possible of the time the drug was taken, for absorption may continue for several hours and an early blood level may not fully reflect the severity of the case. The best guide is serial levels assessed in the light of full clinical knowledge of the patient. A level of 35 mg %, which is above the therapeutic range may be taken as confirming the diagnosis although levels below this may be associated with poisoning and a level of 70 mg % or over indicates that the case is serious.

The key to treatment of acute salicylate poisoning is a sense of urgency and speed. As soon as the diagnosis is suspected, blood for salicylate estimation is drawn and the result requested as an emergency. Gastric aspiration and lavage should then be performed regardless of when the drug was ingested. Provided no contraindication exists, forced alkaline diuresis is started. Acute salicylate poisoning is the one common condition in which this treatment is extremely successful, and it is possible to halve the blood level in as little as eight hours. By this time the blood salicylate level should be available and can be taken into consideration with the time of ingestion, dose stated to have been taken (often exaggerated), history of vomiting, amount recovered by lavage and the clinical state of the patient in assessing whether the diuresis needs to be continued and if so at what rate. In young conscious patients it is not usually necessary to catheterize the bladder unless the case is serious.

If the case is potentially serious with a blood level of over 70 mg % or over 50 mg % where the drug was ingested within four hours of the estimation then blood gases should be estimated as a baseline and a guide to treatment. It has been stated that adult patients frequently are in a state of alkalaemia and it has previously been considered dangerous to subject such patients to an alkaline regime. However, evidence now exists that this is not the case and the benefits of forced alkaline diuresis should not be denied to the severly poisoned case on the grounds that the initial pH is above 7·4. Such cases of course should be carefully observed. The prothrombin time should be estimated and if elevated, Vitamin K, 10 mg, given intravenously. The blood glucose should be estimated and if necessary serially monitored. Hypoglycaemia may require intravenous glucose administration or if diabetes is precipitated, this will require appropriate treatment.

Most severe cases of salicylate poisoning are dehydrated, from hyperpyrexia, sweating, hyperventilation and vomiting and correction of this is a matter of urgency. Hyperpyrexia should be treated with tepid sponging and vomiting with antiemetics.

Special Circumstances. Where the case is serious and forced alkaline diuresis would normally be undertaken but some contra-indication exists, then peritoneal dialysis should be started right away. Haemodialysis should be considered for acutely ill patients with very high blood levels but it is often more important to initiate speedy treatment with forced diuresis or peritoneal dialysis than to waste several hours attempting to arrange facilities for haemodialysis. In the event it is wise to do both. If metabolic acidosis is severe, give immediate correction with 8·4% sodium bicarbonate intravenously. This solution contains 1 mEq of bicarbonate in 1 ml and the dose should be estimated from the calculated ECF deficit. Close monitoring of blood gases is essential. Exchange transfusions may be necessary in small children in whom forced diuresis should be monitored with great care and of course under complete supervision by the Paediatrician.

POISONING BY ANTIDEPRESSANTS

TRICYCLIC ANTIDEPRESSANTS

This group of drugs is now being prescribed with increasing frequency both in adults for depressive illness and also in children when they are prescribed for nocturnal enuresis. They are a common cause of poisoning, constituting 10 per cent of adult admissions for self poisoning. Examples include amitriptyline (Tryptizol), imipramine (Tofranil) and protriptyline (Concordin).

Presentation

The clinical picture of tricyclic poisoning is fairly characteristic and often enables the diagnosis to be suspected on purely

250

clinical grounds. The drugs have a complicated action on the nervous system with varying amounts of central excitation and depression and also possess peripheral anticholinergic and sympathomimetic activity.

There may be initial restlessness and excitement usually leading on to drowsiness or coma. Myoclonus or other involuntary movements may be present and may herald convulsions. Bilateral pyramidal signs with clonus and extensor plantar responses are common. The pupils are usually widely dilated and respond poorly to light and this is often an important diagnostic clue. Anticholinergic effects elsewhere lead to dry mouth, retention of urine and paralytic ileus.

Temperature regulation is upset with either hypo or hyperthermia and respiration is usually depressed to a variable degree.

The effects on cardiovascular function are important. Sinus tachycardia from vagal block is common but so are dysrhythmias of varying kinds. Multifocal ventricular ectopics, ventricular tachycardia or fibrillation and varying degrees of atrio-ventricular block and bundle branch block all occur. There is also a direct depressant action on myocardial function, with inverted T waves in the ECG which may combine with dysrhythmias to produce hypotension and shock.

Fortunately this frightening picture is somewhat mitigated by the short duration of action of this group of drugs. Absorption from the gastro-intestinal tract is good and the drugs are rapidly metabolized in the liver. Because of this, it is unusual for cases not to be improving after twenty-four hours, but hallucinations, insomnia and other features of hypomania may occur for one to two days after recovery of consciousness and death from late cardiac arrhythmia is well recognized.

Diagnosis. The clinical picture of altered conscious level, dilated pupils, unequal or unreactive to light, fits and pyramidal signs in tricyclic poisoning must be differentiated most carefully from organic neurological disease. Subarachnoid haemorrhage, intracerebral infarction or haemorrhage, trauma, hypoglycaemia and hepatic failure are some of the diagnoses that must be considered and the evidence on which the diagnosis of poisoning rests must be carefully reviewed. A similar picture may be seen in 'Mandrax' poisoning also but usually the clinical course of this poisoning is much more prolonged.

The blood levels of tricyclic antidepressants are low and there is much protein binding. Estimation is difficult and although facilities for measurement in urine are greater, chemical estimation only aids in confirming the diagnosis (usually retrospectively) and not in assessing prognosis or treatment.

Treatment. Treatment rests on intensive supportive therapy. Gastric aspiration may be undertaken within three hours of ingestion but forced diuresis is of no value as renal excretion is minimal. Peritoneal or haemodialysis are likewise not indicated as blood levels are low and protein binding is considerable.

Intensive support follows the general lines indicated. In addition all patients should be on continuous ECG monitoring in view of the propensity to arrhythmias. Sinus tachycardia needs no treatment but ventricular ectopics should be suppressed with lignocaine if more than six per minute. Metacholine or pyridostigmine may be used if routine anti-arrhythmic drugs fail. Occasionally heart block may necessitate a temporary transvenous pacemaker. Hypotension in the absence of arrhythmia should be treated as outlined under barbiturate poisoning but added care should be taken with pressor drugs because of their dysrhythmic potency.

If myoclonus develops, it is wise to treat this with diazepam 5 mg intravenously to forestall the appearance of generalized convulsions which themselves may respond to this drug by intravenous infusion or phenobarbitone. Occasionally thiopentone by infusion and mechanical ventilation are required.

MONO-AMINE OXIDASE INHIBITORS (MAOI)

These drugs are either hydrazines such as phenelzine (Nardil) or non-hydrazines such as tranylcypromine (Parnate). Nowadays these drugs are used much less but nevertheless the effects of poisoning are occasionally seen and are usually dramatic. The great danger with this group of drugs is not usually overdosage but untoward effects caused by interaction with other drugs or foodstuffs.

MAOI may potentiate the effects of opiates, barbiturates

and all centrally depressant drugs including alcohol. Insulin and sulphonylureas may be potentiated. Dangerous effects may follow use with tricyclic antidepressants, anticholinergics or anti-hypertensive drugs, and practically all centrally acting agents. Foodstuffs containing tyramine such as cheese, broad beans, marmite, pickled herring or chianti may precipitate hypertensive crises as may L-Dopa.

Presentation

A 'hypertensive' type of reaction may occur following release by drugs of accumulated noradrenaline in nerve endings. The effects are variable. There may be cerebral excitation, headache, convulsions and coma with hyperpyrexia and greatly elevated blood pressure following use with sympathomimetics, foodstuffs, or guanethidine or other hypotensive agents which are antagonized. On the other hand coma, respiratory depression and hypotension may follow use with phenothiazines or opiate analgesics such as pethidine. This is a potentiation phenomenon. The diagnosis may be missed by failing to think of this group of drugs. MAOI are occasionally taken in overdosage alone when the features of cerebral stimulation are prominent. Restlessness, convulsions and hyperpyrexia may exist with either a low or high blood pressure.

Treatment. Supportive treatment is the rule. Hypertensive crisis is best treated with phentolamine mesylate (Rogitine) 5 mg i.v. which is a quick-acting α-adrenergic blocking agent. Ganglion blocking agents are unreliable and may cause the blood pressure to rise. Hypotension should be treated by posture alone or plasma volume expanders such as dextran. Sympathomimetic drugs are dangerous and unreliable. Convulsions should be treated routinely with phenobarbitone or valium. Forced diuresis and peritoneal dialysis are of no value but haemodialysis is reported to be of benefit in severe cases.

LITHIUM CARBONATE

This is used in the treatment of manic depressive psychosis. The features of overdosage are reminiscent of uncontrolled diabetes with thirst, polyuria and vomiting leading to drowsiness. Convulsions may occur. Supportive therapy and forced alkaline diuresis should be employed.

POISONING WITH NON-BARBITURATE CENTRAL DEPRESSANT DRUGS

A very large number of drugs with sedative, tranquillizing or hypnotic properties are now on the market. In general, poisoning with these agents is treated by intensive supportive care but reference to particular agents may be made.

PHENOTHIAZINES

This group of 'major' tranquillizers is used largely for psychotic illness. They are well absorbed but blood levels are low and half life is very prolonged due to an active entero-hepatic circulation.

Presentation

The patient is usually drowsy or unconscious. Extra pyramidal features are common with Parkinsonism, involuntary movements and sometimes a curious state of restless agitation (akathisia). Fits may occur. The blood pressure is usually low due largely to the adrenergic blocking action of these drugs although arrhythmias do occur. Hypothermia is common. Respiratory depression is very uncommon but may occur. Urine specimens should be saved for chromatographic screening as a diagnostic aid.

Treatment. This is supportive. Extrapyramidal features and convulsions may respond to benztropine B-(Cogentin) 1—2 mg slowly intravenously before routine therapy.

DIAZEPINS

Drugs in this group include -diazepam (Valium), nitrazepam (Mogadon) and chloridiazepoxide (Librium). Acute poisoning is common but clinical features are not usually severe. Depression of consciousness is usually not profound and the patient is often

254

drowsy or disorientated. Dysarthria, nystagmus and ataxia combine to produce a picture very similar to alcohol intoxication. Hypotension may occur but significant respiratory depression is unusual. Treatment is supportive only and adjunctive measures are not effective.

MEPROBAMATE

This drug is used more commonly in the USA. Features of overdosage are similar to diazepins except that respiratory depression, hypotension and hypothermia are more common. Blood levels may be helpful in diagnosis, a level below 5 mg % is usually consistent with consciousness and levels of 20 mg % are consistent with deep coma. However, as with many drugs, marked tolerance may occur in habitual users which reduces the value of the test. Treatment is supportive in the vast majority of cases although haemodialysis should be considered in severe cases.

'MANDRAX' POISONING

Mandrax consists of the anti-histamine diphenhydramine and the hypnotic methaqualone and is extensively prescribed as a hypnotic. It is a common cause of poisoning and a dangerous one, the main deleterious effects being ascribable to the methaqualone component.

Presentation

The clinical features are similar to those seen in tricyclic poisoning but the effects are usually more prolonged. Deep coma is usual and may be combined with bilateral pyramidal signs, fits and even papilloedema. Clearly organic neurological disease must be carefully considered in the differential diagnosis. Respiratory depression occurs but is not usually severe. In the cardiovascular system, there may be variable dysrhythmias and ECG changes and myocardial depression can lead to hypotension and acute pulmonary oedema. Blood levels of methaqualone can be measured and levels of 3 mg % are usually considered dangerous, though much higher levels may be encountered.

Treatment. Treatment is by supportive therapy. All patients should have an ECG monitor and close observation is essential. Patients may remain comatose for three to four days and in these circumstances the provision of intensive supportive care is of the utmost importance. Serial chest X-rays may be necessary to detect early bronchopneumonia or partial lobar collapse which should be treated energetically and great attention must be given to fluid and electrolyte balance. Fits should be treated energetically and the appearance of myoclonus regarded as a premonitory sign. Haemodialysis has been used for severe cases but its effectiveness should be regarded as not proven. Forced diuresis is contraindicated due to the danger of precipitating pulmonary oedema. In any case only 2% of unchanged methaqualone is excreted in the urine.

GLUTETHIMIDE (DORIDEN)

Though not as commonly taken as 'Mandrax', poisoning with this drug is dangerous and the clinical picture worthy of especial note. Glutethimide is well absorbed after oral administration. It is fat soluble which probably accounts for its prolonged action. Metabolism is predominantly hepatic.

Presentation

Coma is usual but characteristically is prolonged and fluctuating in severity. The patient seems to recover only to lapse again and become deeply unconscious. The pupils may be unequal or dilated and unresponsive to light as seen in tricyclic poisoning and due to an anticholinergic effect. Respiratory depression and hypotension may both be severe, and respiratory arrest is common. Papilloedema and cerebral oedema with pyramidal signs may be found. Blood levels may be measured and a level of 3 mg % may be regarded as indicating severe poisoning.

Treatment. Treatment is supportive but attention should be given to certain aspects. Gastric lavage should be done if the dose has been ingested within three hours and it has been suggested that the addition of castor oil in equal quantities to the lavage fluid may help to prevent further absorption of the fat soluble drug.

It is important to monitor respiratory function closely and continuously, for respiratory depression may fluctuate. Blood gas estimations should be performed and acidosis corrected. Mechanical ventilation may be needed and facilities for this should be readily to hand. In the presence of papilloedema, pyramidal signs or acute respiratory arrest, it is wise to give an intravenous infusion of 200 ml of 10% mannitol to combat cerebral oedema. Forced diuresis and peritoneal dialysis are not useful and haemodialysis is not of proven value. It is important to remember that the course of glutethimide poisoning may be prolonged and fluctuant and intensive therapy should not be terminated until the patient has clearly improved and the improvement been maintained for several hours.

ALCOHOL (ETHYL ALCOHOL, ETHANOL)

The effects of acute alcohol intoxication in a mild form are too well known to repeat here, but when taken in large quantities, ethyl alcohol produces a dangerous poisoning. A blood level of 300 mg % or greater may be associated with deep coma and respiratory depression. Because alcohol is consumed socially, the stomach may be full at the time of poisoning and there is a correspondingly greater risk of vomiting and aspiration of vomitus into the lungs.

Treatment. The stomach should be aspirated dry whenever the dose was taken. Full supportive therapy is needed. Antiemetics are given for uncontrolled vomiting. Blood sugar should be estimated because hypoglycaemia may occur particularly in children (accidental poisoning). Peritoneal and haemodialysis are both effective in very severe cases.

In alcoholics admitted to hospital and deprived of alcohol or admitted after a period of abstention, convulsions may occur either isolated or together with the delirium tremens withdrawal state. This may be encountered during recovery from acute alcoholic poisoning. The clinical picture is of agitation, insomnia and restlessness. The patient acutely tremulous and hallucinated, picking at the bed clothes, unable to relax and with secondary

257

delusions. Treatment is by chlorpromazine 100 mg i.m. 4-hourly until sedation is achieved and parentrovite 2 ampoules daily intravenously for ten days. Fits should be treated with diazepam or phenobarbitone. Alcohol should not be given in treatment.

METHYLALCOHOL

Methanol poisoning is seen mostly in down and outs who drink methylated spirits but it can be taken accidentally. The clinical features are variable depression of consciousness, severe vomiting, visual impairment sometimes with papillitis, headache and gasping (Kussmaul) respiration.

Treatment. The clinical features are due to a severe metabolic acidosis which develops because the oxidative metabolism of methanol leads to the formation of formic acid. Visual disturbances result from acute optic neuritis. Full supportive therapy including gastric lavage should be given. Blood gases should be estimated and immediate correction of the acidosis made with 8·4% sodium bicarbonate solution intravenously. Because methanol and ethanol share the same oxidative enzyme systems, giving ethyl alcohol will slow the rate of metabolism of methyl alcohol by substrate competition. 30 ml of absolute ethyl alcohol diluted in 100 ml water should be given orally and repeated 4-hourly for several days. In a severe case where visual changes are found initially or supervene later, the patient should be haemodialyzed.

OPIATE NARCOTICS

This group includes morphine, heroin, codeine and dihydro-codeine (DF 118). Overdosage with these drugs is met largely in two situations, clinical overdosage or misuse (for instance in a patient with diminished respiratory reserve) and in addicts. The clinical features are similar and include coma, pin-point (but equal and reactive) pupils, hypotension and profound respiratory depression. If the patient is addicted, evidence may be found on examination. Needle tracks in the arms with multiple scars, infected areas and thrombosed veins. There may be marked weight loss or anaemia or jaundice and a generally dishevelled air. It is now illegal (without special licence) to supply heroin to an addict, and this must be remembered.

Treatment. A specific pharmacological antagonist exists to the opiates. Nalorphine is related to morphine and has equivalent analgesic activity. Antagonism is not simple and varies for different actions being most prominent for respiratory and circulatory depression. It may dilate contracted pupils and may produce a withdrawal state in addicts. In addition to full supportive therapy Nalorphine hydrobromide 15 mg should be given intravenously and repeated at intervals of 15—30 minutes until the patient is recovered. Respiration should be closely monitored and facilities for mechanical ventilation be always available. If the patient is addicted and has taken an overdose, withdrawal features may be anticipated on recovery. These may include vasomotor rhinorrhoea, sweating and shivering, passing on to increasing agitation, vomiting, abdominal pain and shock. Treatment is by sedation and methadone 20 mg at repeated intervals.

ANTICHOLINERGICS (INCLUDING ATROPINE, HOMATROPINE, HYOSCINE AND PROPANTHELINE) AND ANTIHISTAMINIC DRUGS

These are considered together because the clinical features and treatment of acute poisoning by them are similar. Antihistamine drugs commonly have strong anticholinergic effects. Both groups of drugs are commonly well absorbed and metabolized mainly in the liver.

Presentation

Effects on the nervous system are a variable mixture of depression and excitation. Variable depression of conscious level occurs or an agitated and tremulous state with disorientation, hallucinations and convulsions. The pupils may be dilated, unequal and non-reactive to light. Failure of accommodation, urinary retention, dry mouth and paralytic ileus complete the picture of parasympathetic blockade. Hyperpyrexia may occur and cardiac dysrhythmias also. Depression of respiration may be fatal.

259

Treatment. Full supportive care is given. Excitement and hallucinations should be treated with phenobarbitone 100–200 mg intramuscularly repeated before convulsions develop.

Neostigmine may reverse the peripheral anticholinergic effects but does not affect the more serious central involvement. Forced diuresis and dialysis regimes are not effective.

OTHER DRUGS

Occasionally other hypnotic or sedative drugs are taken in over-dosage. These include methylpentynol (Oblivon), ethchlorvynol or drugs of the chloral group (chloral, triclofos or dichloral-phenazone). In general, treatment is by supportive therapy and the clinical picture is neither severe nor has any specific features. Mild poisoning resembles acute alcoholic intoxication. Chloral can cause gastritis, hepatic and renal damage.

SYMPATHOMIMETICS

The amphetamines are the most common drugs in this group taken in overdosage. The reason for this is their use as stimulants by the young (purple hearts, black bombers, etc.). The drugs produce tolerance and therefore the dose required to produce the clinical picture of poisoning varies enormously. They are well absorbed orally and about half the dose is excreted unchanged in the urine, though this is increased if the urine is made acid. The clinical features of amphetamine poisoning are shared to a great extent by other sympathomimetics such as ephedrine.

Presentation

The patient is often young and may deny consumption of the drug. Restlessness, hypermobility and agitation are prominent, going on to wild excitement and delirium and perhaps convulsions and coma. There is marked pallor, sweating and tremor and the reflexes are very brisk. A common complaint is of palpitation, and severe headache is usual. Cardiac arrhythmias are common and both tachycardias and atrio-ventricular block with ventricular extrasystoles occur. Angina or myocardial infarction may be precipitated and the patient may go into severe shock. Vomiting, abdominal pain and gastrointestinal haemorrhage may occur.

With drugs such as isoprenaline which stimulate β receptors only, the central effects are less common but the cardiac manifestations may be severe.

Treatment. The diagnosis and management are essentially clinical as blood levels may vary enormously owing to tolerance. Supportive therapy should be full and include continuous ECG monitoring. Cardiac arrhythmias may respond to practolol, a β-blocking drug, 100 mg b.d. orally or 5–10 mg slowly intravenously according to their nature. Rogitine 5 mg intravenously, an α adrenergic blocker may be helpful but often dysrhythmias are bizarre. If atrioventricular block occurs, atropine should be tried. The patient should be sedated with diazepam or chlorpromazine, oxygen therapy and adequate fluid should be maintained. Forced acid diuresis should be employed in severe cases and haemodialysis may be of benefit.

DOMESTIC SUBSTANCES

A variety of toxic substances are included in household preparations such as pesticides, certain cosmetics, polishes, solvents and disinfectants. Poisoning with these substances is more often truly accidental and frequently involves children. A wide variety of proprietary products exists and only some of the more dangerous are described. It is advisable to contact the nearest 'Poisons Centre' immediately if any doubt exists as to the nature or toxic properties of any household substance taken.

PARAQUAT POISONING

Paraquat is a herbicide that acts by inhibiting photosynthesis. It is available in a liquid form as a 20% solution (gramoxone) which is only available to farmers and horticulturalists and also as solid granules (5%) — Weedol, which can be bought without licence for home gardening. Fatalities are more common with the concentrated form but occur with both. Often the solution has been put into a different bottle and is taken by accident.

Public education to the enormous danger of paraquat must continue.

Clinical Features

The initial features are common to any corrosive poison, and consist of burns to the upper gastrointestinal tract, giving a pharyngitis and oesophagitis. It is the later features that are dangerous and as there is often a delay of several days before these appear and the patient may be relatively well in this time, it is of the utmost importance that the patient is not discharged early.

Hepatitis and acute renal failure are two of the later sequelae but both these are potentially reversible with adequate therapy and the really serious complication is a progressive fibrosing alveolitis which presents as progressive dyspnoea, cyanosis and basal râles in the chest. Bilateral shadowing in the lung fields appears on chest X-ray and the pulmonary function tests show a progressive deterioration in gas transfer (D_{CO}).

Treatment. It is essential to treat this poisoning energetically from the outset. Gastric lavage should be undertaken. Forced diuresis should be started with careful watch on renal function, and haemodialysis should probably be performed where the case is serious or renal damage has occurred. Full supportive therapy is essential and the patient must be observed in hospital for at least ten days however mild the poisoning. Unfortunately there does not seem to be any means of halting the progress of the pulmonary lesion once established. Steroids do not seem particularly effective but should be tried. Pulmonary transplantation may be indicated in progressive cases but it is not certain that the pulmonary damage does not affect the transplanted lung, even if the paraquat has been totally removed.

CHLORATE

Sodium chlorate is used as a weed-killer. Vomiting, abdominal pain and diarrhoea may be followed by acute renal and hepatic failure. Methaemoglobinaemia and severe haemolysis occur. Supportive therapy is supplemented by ascorbic acid 1 g intra-

venously for severe methaemoglobinaemia. Haemodialysis or
peritoneal dialysis may be helpful particularly when renal failure
supervenes.

INSECTICIDES

DDT

This is the most widely used of all insecticides. In general there
is a wide safety margin used judiciously but lipid solvents can
increase absorption from the gut or skin. Symptoms begin 2 to
3 hours after ingestion and toxicity is largely confined to the
nervous system. Paraesthesiae of the legs and tremors of the eye-
lids lead on to ataxia, convulsions and coma. Death may ensue
from respiratory failure or ventricular fibrillation, but otherwise
recovery is not prolonged. Treatment is supportive with continuous ECG and respiratory monitoring.

ORGANOPHOSPHOROUS INSECTICIDES (PARATHION, DYFLOS)

These substances act by inhibiting chloninesterase almost irrevers-
ibly and are extremely dangerous. The clinical picture is of
gross parasympathetic overactivity. Anorexia, vomiting and restless confusion with colicky abdominal pain and diarrhoea are
prominent early on. The skin is cold and sweaty and excess
salivation occurs. After several hours muscle twitching, weakness and convulsions occur, there is severe bronchospasm,
cyanosis and pulmonary oedema, and respiratory arrest is
common. The heart rate is slow and hypotension and shock may
occur.

Treatment. The most common route of entry is through the
skin. Contaminated clothes are removed and the skin washed
with alcohol. Full supportive therapy is commenced with
facilities for mechanical ventilation closely to hand. The patient
should be fully atropinized and kept so for at least twenty-four
hours. Large doses may be required, 1 mg every fifteen minutes.
As soon as the diagnosis is suspected, steps should be taken
to obtain the antidote, pralidoxine (PAM). The address of the

nearest supply should be obtainable from the Poisons Information Service. Pralidoxine is a specific reactivator of cholinesterase and is given intravenously in doses of 1—2 g and repeated as necessary. Barbiturates, opiates, aminophylline, reserpine, phenothiazines and depolarizing neuromuscular blocking agents are all potentiated and great care is needed in the use of any of these agents. Fits should be controlled with thiopentone and mechanical ventilation may well be needed. The blood level of cholinesterase can be measured serially and the patient rested until it is 70 per cent of normal which may take many weeks.

PHENOLIC INSECTICIDES AND WEED KILLERS

Dinitrophenol and related compounds (dinitro-orthocresol) uncouple oxidative phosphorylation and lead to a large increase in the heat production of the body. Poisoning usually results from skin staining (yellow) or inhalation during crop spraying.

Presentation

The skin is stained yellow. If taken orally there is a corrosive action. There is central stimulation with agitation, confusion, convulsions and finally coma. The body temperature is usually raised, and sweating in proportion to the dose and thirst are prominent. Dyspnoea and tachycardia complete the picture, although hepatic and renal damage may both occur as complications.

Treatment. Treatment is supportive. Contaminated clothing is removed and the skin washed. Hyperpyrexia should be treated with fans and tepid sponging and chlorpromazine may be helpful. Dehydration may need urgent correction.

Phenols. Phenol (carbolic acid) or related substances such as lysol or cresol are used as disinfectants and are general protoplasmic poisons and corrosives. When ingested, necrotic burns of the pharynx and oesophagus may result, which are frequently painless, but the incidence of severe corrosion is surprisingly low. Systemic effects are serious however. Profound coma, hypothermia, shock and respiratory failure are common and renal failure may also occur. Serious effects can follow cutaneous absorption. Treatment is supportive. Gastric lavage with water should be undertaken with care. Intravenous infusion of sodium bicarbonate may help though severe acidosis is not well documented. There is a small risk of stricture of the oesophagus developing later.

ORGANIC SOLVENTS AND CLEANING SUBSTANCES

CARBON TETRACHLORIDE

This organic solvent is still used as a cleaning substance. It is extremely toxic when taken orally, producing coma with circulatory and respiratory collapse followed (if the patient survives) by severe hepatic and renal disease. Treatment is by full supportive care.

A wide variety of common domestic products, including many solvents, cleaners and polishes, contain toxic substances. Some of these and their main effects and treatment are tabulated.

HYPOCHLORITE POISONING

Household bleaches and some disinfectants contain sodium hypochlorite from which free chlorine may be liberated in the stomach by the action of gastric acid. Local corrosive action and pulmonary oedema following inhalation of chlorine result. Treatment is supportive with gastric aspiration and lavage with 1% sodium thiosulphate. Pulmonary oedema should be treated with steroids.

OXALIC ACID POISONING

Oxalic acid is found in metal polishes, bleaches, and rust and ink eradicators. Its toxicity is high with an initial corrosive action on gastrointestinal mucosa leading to severe vomiting, diarrhoea and shock. Systemic effects follow and result from hypo-calcaemia following the formation of insoluble calcium oxalate.

Drugs	*Product*	*Effects*	*Treatment*
Aromatic Hydrocarbons (Benzene, Toluene, Xylol)	Inks Leather dyes Nail polish Nail polish remover	GIT Irritant Pulmonary oedema CNS Inebriation Fits. Coma.	Supportive Monitor ECG Ascorbic Acid i.v.
Petroleum distillates	Kerosene Metal polish Shoe polish Solvents Insect repellants	Haemorrhagic alveolitis CNS Depression	Supportive No lavage Avoid pulmonary aspiration Steroids
Toxic alcohols (butyl, isopropryl)	Solvents After-shave Nail polish Floor polish	GIT irritant Inebriation → Coma Respiratory failure	Supportive Correct acidosis Haemodialysis
Turpentine	Oil of turpentine	GIT irritant Pulmonary oedema Coma	Supportive
Naphthalene	Air deodorants Moth balls	GIT irritant Haemolysis Jaundice Renal failure	Supportive Alkalinize urine Steroids Transfusion
Ethylene Glycol	Antifreeze	Inebriation → Coma Respiratory collapse CVS collapse Acidosis Hypocalcaemia Renal failure	Supportive Calcium i.v. Correct acidosis Ethyl alcohol Haemodialysis

Toxic effects and treatment of poisoning by some common domestic products.

Tetany, fits, coma and cardiac arrest are common. Treatment is supportive. Gastric lavage is dangerous but hypocalcaemia must be controlled with intravenous infusion of calcium gluconate in 500 ml of saline over four hours monitored by hourly Trousseau tests for latent tetany and frequent serum calcium estimations. The dose of calcium given is determined from the calculated ECF deficit. Dehydration must be avoided as calcium oxalate may precipitate in the kidney and late renal failure is well recognized.

PHOSPHORUS POISONING

Severe phosphorus poisoning has resulted from ingestion of rat poisons. Initial vomiting and diarrhoea (which may be luminescent) may proceed to shock or an asymptomatic period of up to several days. The third or systemic phase is of massive vomiting and diarrhoea with haematemesis, generalized bleeding, hepatic and renal failure, and coma. Treatment is supportive. Contaminated clothing is removed and gastric lavage undertaken. Vitamin K or fresh blood transfusion may be required for bleeding due to hypoprothrombinaemia. Acidosis must be corrected with sodium bicarbonate.

Mild phosphorus poisoning can result if young children ingest the heads of the 'strike anywhere' type of match which contains phosphorus on the match head. Usually mild vomiting and diarrhoea result but liver damage may occur. Treatment is supportive.

POISONING BY INHALED GASES

CARBON MONOXIDE POISONING

The usual sources of this substance are coal gas and motor exhaust fumes. Carbon monoxide has an affinity for haemoglobin three hundred times greater than oxygen. The formation of carboxyhaemoglobin results in hypoxaemia and consequent tissue hypoxia. It is an extremely dangerous form of poisoning with the highest mortality of any form of poisoning in adults.

Presentation

The difficulty is grading the severity of the case for deterioration can take place rapidly. In the nervous system the effects are due to hypoxia with consequent secondary cerebral oedema. Mental changes are prominent, restlessness and confusion may dominate the picture or may pass on sometimes quickly to deep coma which may be irreversible. Bilateral pyramidal signs are common and papilloedema may occur. There may be a high fever, and sudden respiratory failure may occur. The neurological changes are not only temporary. Permanent sequelae may result; intellectual impairment or hemiplegia. On the other hand, initial changes may clear up to be followed weeks later by permanent damage. Parkinsonism may occur or a cerebellar syndrome or any degree of impairment of higher functions.

Because of the hypoxaemia the myocardium suffers. ECG changes of T-wave inversion indicating ischaemia occur in the majority of severe cases but damage may be more severe, particularly in those with pre-existing ischaemic heart disease or the elderly, and myocardial infarction, dysrhythmias and shock are all reported. Shock may be worsened by gastrointestinal bleeding, probably from ischaemia. Classically the skin and mucosae are coloured bright cherry pink in carbon monoxide poisoning due to the colour of carboxyhaemoglobin but the change is in fact only seen in very severely poisoned patients, many of whom come to post mortem. In most patients who survive, this is not seen.

Treatment. Speed is absolutely essential and no case, however seemingly mild, should be treated lightly. The patient must immediately be removed from the scene of contamination. This will, of course, usually have been done by the time the patient is seen in hospital but is worth emphasizing for the education of ancillary staff such as ambulance drivers who may be called to see the patient at home. Oxygen therapy should be commenced at once in the ambulance if the diagnosis is clear as it very often is. It is much more important to give this early treatment than to insist on a proper medical opinion. As high a concentration of oxygen in the inhaled air as is possible should be achieved and the combination of an MRC mask and nasal spectacles from two cylinders of 100% oxygen is a quick way to achieve this. The use of a mixture of 95% oxygen and 5% carbon dioxide has been recommended for its respiratory stimulant effect. While this may be helpful in some patients, if respiratory depression exists, it is much more important to measure ventilatory function and institute mechanical aid if necessary.

After the institution of oxygen therapy as quickly as possible, the patient is given full supportive care. Continuous ECG monitoring is necessary and complete bed rest for several days should be enforced whatever the age of the patient. Bilateral

268

pyramidal signs, deteriorating conscious level, hyperventilation, papilloedema or any other evidence of raised intracranial pressure should be treated promptly with an infusion of 200 ml of 10% mannitol, repeated if necessary in four hours.

Hyperbaric oxygen therapy should be considered for severe cases, but is probably not essential. Carboxyhaemoglobin levels fall rapidly once the patient is removed from contamination and oxygen therapy is started, and because of the delay in instituting hyperbaric therapy (even if a unit is available) the advantages are largely theoretical.

The measurement of carboxyhaemoglobin levels in blood is important to confirm the diagnosis but on no account should treatment await the result. As stated, levels fall quickly and therefore may not constitute a reliable criterion of the severity of the case. By the time blood is taken, the level may be low but severe secondary hypoxic damage may still ensue.

CYANIDE POISONING

Cyanide poisoning usually occurs by the inhalation of hydrocyanic acid gas released inadvertently from the action of strong acids on cyanide salts. It may occur in the stomach after the ingestion of cyanide salts. Cyanide acts as an inhibitor of cytochrome oxidase and hence inhibits oxidative metabolism at cellular level. It is one of the most dangerous and rapidly acting of all poisons.

Presentation

The patient rapidly loses consciousness with dilated pupils and areflexia. Respiratory and cardiovascular depression are both profound but cyanosis is absent. The patient may smell of bitter almonds. Sometimes, if only minimal poisoning has occurred, there may be a promonitory stage with nausea and salivation, confusion and dyspnoea before coma appears.

Treatment. In any case, the speed with which treatment is commenced is the most important factor determining the outcome. It is essential that the necessary drugs are available in a locked cupboard in the Casualty Department and on the Intensive Therapy Unit. Several drugs are used. Nitrites induce

269

the formation of methaemoglobin which then competes with cytochrome oxidase for the cyanide radicle. About thirty per cent of the circulating haemoglobin must be so changed. An ampoule of amyl nitrite should be inhaled immediately while an injection of sodium nitrite (10 ml of 3% solution) is drawn up and injected intravenously slowly. Respiration will usually be severely depressed and the institution of mechanical ventilation at this stage is necessary. High oxygen concentrations should be given.

Next sodium thiosulphate should be injected intravenously (25 ml of 50% solution injected over fifteen minutes). This converts cyanide into non-toxic thiocyanate. In addition, the stomach should be aspirated and lavage carried out with 5% sodium thiosulphate. Cobalt acetate (Kelocyanor) can also be used, 300 mg being injected intravenously very slowly, and hydroxycobalamine (Neocytamen) 1 mg intravenously may chelate cyanide to form cyanocobalamin and should be given. If recovery is achieved by this emergency regime, then full supportive care is necessary for at least three days, preferably with ECG monitoring.

IRRITANT GASES

Irritant gases may be inhaled from time to time. Ammonia, hydrochloric acid and formaldehyde tend to produce an acute rhinitis, tracheitis or bronchitis only but chlorine and sulphur dioxide commonly produce a chemical pneumonitis as well. Nitrogen dioxide is dangerous as the initial irritant effect is minimal but is followed after an asymptomatic period of up to two days by a progressive alveolitis with pulmonary oedema and respiratory and circulatory collapse. Treatment is supportive but steroids should be given in all forms of chemical pneumonitis with pulmonary oedema and a careful watch kept on ventilatory function and respiratory toilet.

NATURAL POISONS

BOTULISM
Presentation

Botulism is caused entirely by the ingestion of pre-formed toxin of Clostridium Botulinum in foodstuffs. The toxins, of which

270

there are six immunological types, A, B, C, D, E and F, act by impairing the release of acetylcholine at all cholinergic synapses. They are relatively heat stable and will resist boiling for up to ten minutes. Home canning of foods, which are then stored under conditions in which contained spores of Clostridium Botulinum may germinate and produce toxin is responsible for most cases. Type A gives probably the most serious illness with a mortality of 60—70 per cent. Type E is most often contracted from fish foods, and as this strain does not produce proteolytic enzymes, the food does not smell or taste 'off'.

Botulism may be a relatively mild illness or may be fulminant with death within hours. Symptoms normally commence from 12 to 36 hours after ingestion of the contaminated food but may be delayed for up to fourteen days. The patient may initially complain of neurological symptoms such as diplopia, dysarthria and dysphagia with signs of cranial nerve paresis progressing to general muscular paralysis. The reflexes are usually preserved and there is no sensory deficit. Respiratory failure is common and may progress rapidly. Particularly in Type E poisoning, gastrointestinal symptoms may be prominent and may delay recognition of neurological signs. Vomiting and abdominal pain with constipation may lead to a diagnosis of intestinal obstruction. Urinary retention, dry mouth and dilated pupils can suggest atropine poisoning. Characteristically though, the patient's mental state is normal without the central excitatory effect seen in atropine poisoning.

The differential diagnosis also includes myaesthenia gravis and Guillain—Barre syndrome. A Tensilon test may help to exclude the former and the lack of sensory loss the latter. The history of suspect food intake may help but may not be easy to obtain. Food samples should be obtained if possible and may be cultured for Clostridium Botulinum. The toxin may also be identified in food or in the patient's serum by its lethal action in the mouse unprotected by antiserum.

Treatment. The initial and most important part of treatment is supportive. Respiratory failure may be sudden and continuous monitoring of ventilatory function is essential. If deterioration occurs it is probably wise to proceed to tracheostomy early as respiratory paralysis may persist for up to two months.

271

Mechanical ventilation may be required for the whole of this time and therefore most careful respiratory toilet and physiotherapy is necessary. Bulbar paralysis may make tube feeding or parenteral nutrition necessary and again, because the illness may be prolonged, special care in the provision of adequate nutrition is needed. Urinary catheterization may be necessary if the patient develops retention of urine and also phsysiotherapy to paralyzed limbs. Enemas should be given to prevent further absorption of toxin from the colon which may give delayed symptoms.

Specific antisera against each immunological type of toxin exist but there is no cross-protection. Types C and D are not responsible for disease in humans and type F rarely so. The patient should be given the whole dose of antiserum in one injection (after a test dose for horse serum sensitivity) as it persists in the body for thirty days. 100 000 units of bivalent A and B antiserum and 10 000 units of type E antiserum should be given subcutaneously. One-third of these doses should be given to exposed persons who have not as yet developed symptoms.

Antibiotic therapy should be reserved for specific infective complications as there is no evidence that Clostridium Botulinium itself when ingested contributes to the disease. Recently guanidine hydrochloride has been used with some success in botulism. This drug reduces the neuromuscular block produced by the toxins. Therapy which is oral in doses of 15–30 mg per kg per day may have to be prolonged for many weeks. Side effects include hyperexcitability, tremors and gastrointestinal disturbance.

SNAKE BITE

The only poisonous snake indigenous to the United Kingdom is the adder. Its bite is very rarely lethal but may produce severe effects particularly in a small child. The site of the bite is identified by two puncture marks and local effects consist of the signs of acute inflammation spreading for a variable distance from the bite. If a large dose of venom has been injected, then vomiting, abdominal pain and diarrhoea may ensue followed in really severe cases by confusion, shock and respiratory failure.

Treatment is local by immobilizing the involved limb. Hydrocortisone 100 mg intramuscularly is recommended but not the antivenom which may produce dangerous reactions. A venous tourniquet may help stop spread of poison in the short term. Otherwise full supportive treatment is given for complications as they develop, including sedation for anxiety and antibiotics for any superadded infection. Prophylaxis appropriate to the immune status should be given against tetanus.

'MUSHROOM' POISONING

The edible mushrooms may be mistaken for others. The most commonly taken poisonous fungus is Amanita phalloides which is unfortunately extremely toxic. Furthermore, the poison survives cooking.

After the plant is eaten the patient is usually quite well for several hours and the lull may trap the unwary. Then the patient develops all the features of acute cholinergic poisoning due to muscarine in the plant. There is severe intestinal colic with vomiting and diarrhoea. Acute dehydration may occur and even shock. Brachycardia, excessive salivation and bronchial constriction develop with mental changes and respiratory depression. If this is survived the patient may then go on to develop renal failure, acute hepatic necrosis with sometimes profound hypoglycaemia and severe neurological changes with coma.

Treatment. Treatment is full supportive care including treatment of hepatic and renal failure. The stomach should be aspirated. Haemodialysis is indicated if there is evidence early on of hepatic damage and proteinuria. This may forestall the development of more severe changes as after forty-eight hours the toxins are no longer dialysable. Full atropinization is essential in the cholinergic phase. Careful daily checks should be made on urea and electrolytes, blood gases, blood sugar, liver function tests and serum calcium. Dehydration must be watched for early on and corrected. Other fungi are not so poisonous but may present a similar picture.

Other Plants. Cholinergic poisoning is also seen with Aconite (the Monkshood) and the opposite picture of atropine poisoning

273

is seen following ingestion of the Deadly Nightshade (Belladonna). Mistletoe berries are poisonous and give a similar picture to Digoxin overdosage. The patient should be treated accordingly. Elderberry (bark, leaves) and hydrangea poisoning should be treated urgently as for cyanide poisoning.

There are many other poisonous plants in the United Kingdom, Yew, Laburnum, Lupin and Hemlock to name a few. Treatment is supportive with no specific measures. If any doubt exists, the Poisons Information Service should be contacted urgently, as serious effects such as convulsions or respiratory depression may occur.

HEAVY METAL POISONING, ETC.

IRON POISONING

Poisoning with iron salts is important because it is common, particularly affects young children who take the preparations as sweets, and because it is very dangerous.

The patient is usually a small child who an hour or so after ingestion develops acute vomiting and severe abdominal pain. Haematemesis and melaena are common due to corrosive action on the gastric mucosa and gastric perforation may occur. These features may improve, but vigilance should not be relaxed, for further gastrointestinal haemorrhage and acute neurological signs may appear, with fits, loss of consciousness and respiratory and circulatory depression. Later still, hepatitis may develop or chronic strictures in the gastrointestinal tract up to two months after ingestion.

Treatment. Speed is essential. The stomach is immediately aspirated and lavage carried out with desferrioxamine (a chelating agent for iron). Put 0·2 g in each 200 ml aliquot of fluid. After lavage·10 g of desferrioxamine should be left in the stomach.

At the same time 2 g of desferrioxamine should be injected intramuscularly and repeated twelve-hourly. In addition an intravenous infusion of desferrioxamine at 15 mg/kg/hr should be set up. A total dose 80 mg/kg in twenty-four hours by this route is the maximum. It is useful to measure serum iron levels initially and serially to follow improvement. A level above 500 μg % in a child is very dangerous. Treatment is otherwise supportive. Cerebral oedema may respond to mannitol. Shock, respiratory failure, liver failure and fits should be treated according to established practice.

ACUTE LEAD POISONING

This usually follows contamination (either orally or by skin absorption) with organic compounds of lead such as are used in industry (tetraethyl lead). The clinical picture is that of acute gastrointestinal disturbance with an encephalopathy. Vomiting, severe abdominal colic and diarrhoea pass on to fits and coma. A haemolytic crisis may occur and hepatic and renal failure may ensue.

Treatment. The stomach should be aspirated and full supportive care given. The chelating agent, sodium calcium edetate is very effective and should be given intravenously 50 mg/kg total in twenty-four hours as two one-hour infusions, repeated for three days. This is usually effective treatment for the severe abdominal colic but calcium gluconate, atropine or pethidine may still be required. If cerebral oedema is suspected, an infusion of 200 ml 10% mannitol should be given and repeated in four hours if necessary. If the patient has had chronic exposure to lead, d-penicillamine orally 20—40 mg/kg should be started after recovery. Investigations include the serum lead and urinary excretion of lead and coproporphyrin III. A serum lead level above 0·05 mg % makes the diagnosis of acute poisoning.

MERCURY POISONING

Metallic mercury is not absorbed orally but mercurial compounds are. The initial features are of an extremely acute gastrointestinal disturbance often progressing to shock. Hepatic and renal damage and a membranous colitis follow after one to three days. Treatment is full supportive care and BAL given intramuscularly four-hourly at 5 mg/kg for twenty-four hours then 3 mg/kg for a further twenty-four hours then 3 mg/kg

twelve-hourly for seven days. Toxic effects of vomiting, salivation, skin rashes and tachycardia are common and the injections
are painful. These clinical features and also the treatment are
similar in acute arsenical poisoning and BAL should also be used
in treatment of acute gold, chromate and antimony poisoning.

POISONING BY VARIOUS THERAPEUTIC AGENTS

Various drugs used in medical practice may occasionally be
taken in overdosage by accident, clinical miscalculation or
deliberate intent by the patient.

ANTICONVULSANTS

PHENYTOIN

This drug has a prolonged action. Drowsiness, disinhibition and
a marked cerebellar syndrome develop. Treatment is supportive.

PRIMADONE

This should be treated as phenobarbitone overdosage as it is
metabolized to this drug.

SULTHIAME (Ospolot)

Tachypnoea and pyramidal signs are common. Blood gases
should be monitored and supportive therapy given. Forced alkaline
diuresis may be used for severe cases.

ANTIBIOTICS

Acute allergic reactions, anaphylactic shock, exfoliative
dermatitis or the Stevens Johnson syndrome may be
encountered. Treatment is supportive with correction of
dehydration and use of steroids as necessary. Blood dyscrasias
may present with septicaemia, haemorrhage due to low platelet
count or severe anaemias and should be treated appropriately.

ANTICOAGULANTS

If due to oral agents such as warfarin or phenindione, the blood prothrombin time should be measured and if greater than 50 seconds, Vitamin K 20 mg intravenously daily should be given with daily monitoring of the prothrombin time. If overdosage is due to heparin, protamine sulphate 100 mg should be given slowly intravenously. Haemorrhage may require blood transfusion.

DIGOXIN

The drug has a low therapeutic ratio and overdosage is therefore common. Nausea, vomiting and bradycardia are usual but almost any cardiac arrhythmia may be precipitated. Treatment is to stop the drug and monitor the serum potassium closely. If arrhythmias or ventricular ectopic beats are present, continuous ECG monitoring is essential. Hypokalaemia should be corrected urgently either orally or by intravenous infusion. Arrhythmias are treated according to their nature but β-blocking drugs, propranolol and practolol are very useful.

DIURETICS

Powerful new diuretics such as frusemide may produce dangerous dehydration, hyponatraemia and hypokalaemia when taken in excess. Shock may occur and acute gout or diabetes may be precipitated. Treatment is fluid and electrolyte replacement with careful monitoring of serum electrolytes together with other supportive measures as required.

PHENACETIN POISONING

The clinical effects of overdosage with most proprietary preparations containing phenacetin are mostly from the aspirin also contained but phenacetin is a dangerous substance. Chronic poisoning leads to severe renal damage and acute renal failure may occur during acute poisoning. However, cyanosis from

277

methaemoglobinaemia, acute haemolysis, shock, mental changes and hepatic damage are all common features. Treatment is supportive. Ascorbic acid 1 g intravenously slowly or methylene blue should be given if cyanosis is present due to methaemoglobin. Blood glucose should be measured as hypoglycaemia may contribute to the cerebral abnormalities seen. Hepatic and renal failure are treated according to established practice and haemolytic crisis may require steroids. Paracetamol is less dangerous but is, in fact, the active metabolite of phenacetin and poisoning with it presents in a similar fashion.

National Poisons Information Service

LONDON	Guy's Hospital (New Cross Hospital, London, S.E. 14)	01-407 7600
EDINBURGH	Royal Infirmary	031-229 2477
CARDIFF	Cardiff Royal Infirmary	0222 33101
BELFAST	Royal Victoria Hospital	0232 30503
DUBLIN	Jervis Street Hospital	Dublin 45588

FURTHER READING

Goodman, L. S. and Gilman, A. (1970). *The Pharmacological Basis of Therapeutics*, 4th ed., The Macmillan Co., New York.
Matthew, H. and Lawson, A. A. H. (1967). *Treatment of Common Acute Poisonings*, E. and S. Livingstone Ltd.
Gleason, M. N., Gossdin, R. E., Hodge, H. C. and Smith, R. P. (1969). *Clinical Toxicology of Commercial Products*, 3rd ed., The Williams and Wilkins Co., Baltimore.
Laurence, D. R. (1966). *Clinical Pharmacology*, 3rd ed., J. and A. Churchill Ltd., London.
Polson, C. J. and Tattersall, R. N. (1969). *Clinical Toxicology*, Pitman Medical Publishing Co. Ltd., London.

Chapter 9

Parenteral Nutrition

JOANNA SHELDON

INDICATIONS FOR PARENTERAL THERAPY

PLANNING PARENTERAL NUTRITION

PREPARATIONS

1. CARBOHYDRATE

2. FAT

3. PROTEIN

4. VITAMINS

MANAGEMENT OF INFUSIONS

Some thirty years ago, if oral feeding was impossible or inadvisable, we only had saline and glucose solutions with which to feed patients parenterally, and since 1 litre of normal saline and 1 litre of 5% dextrose, which was commonly the daily fluid prescription, provides only 400 calories and no nitrogen, semi-starvation was inevitable. While this may not adversely affect the course of an illness of moderate severity or short duration, severe or prolonged illness, associated with an increased demand for calories and nitrogen, may be very adversely influenced.

279

Today carbohydrate, fat, protein and vitamins can all be supplied parenterally, and adequate nutrition can thus be maintained over long periods.

Parenteral feeding is required if sufficient cannot be provided by mouth or by tube-feeding, when there is otherwise a realistic chance of survival; some of the chief indications for its use are shown in Table I.

INDICATIONS FOR PARENTERAL THERAPY

TABLE I.

1. Pre-operatively in the severly malnourished.
2. Post-operatively:
   (a) If severely malnourished pre-operatively.
   (b) If prolonged inability to feed by mouth is anticipated.
   (c) If oral feeding is delayed beyond 4—5 days by unexpected complications.
3. Severe malabsorption states (e.g. Regional enteritis).
4. Renal failure.
5. Liver failure. (See Chapter 4.)
6. Severe burns.
7. Hyperemesis gravidarum.
8. Some cases of anorexia nervosa.

PRE-OPERATIVE PARENTERAL NUTRITION

Pre-operatively parenteral nutrition is rarely required; but it may be necessary, for example in patients with obstructing lesions of the gastrointestinal tract, including congenital atresias in infants, or in ulcerative colitis and malabsorption states associated with considerable weight loss. Under these circumstances it may be impossible to achieve positive nitrogen balance pre-operatively with an ordinary hospital diet. Nitrogen balance can usually be restored with a 2—5 day period of parenteral feeding supplying 35—40 cals/kg/day (2500—3000 cals/day for a 70 kg adult), and 1·0—1·5 g protein/kg/day (70—100 g protein/day for a 70 kg adult). This helps to reduce the incidence of post-operative complications, because severe malnutrition, with hypo-proteinaemia, is associated with poor wound healing, delayed gastric emptying and reduced intestinal motility, and increased susceptibility to haemorrhagic shock and infection. In addition,

280

liver function may be impaired post-operatively in the mal-nourished, possibly due to reduced liver glycogen.

Post-operative Parenteral Nutrition

Post-operatively, and after trauma, a negative nitrogen balance occurs, which is often tacitly assumed to be an inevitable reaction to injury. However, there is evidence that this increased protein breakdown may be simply the result of an inadequate diet, or of complications of surgery which increase protein cata-bolism, such as fever and sepsis. Thus it has been shown that nitrogen deficits developing during the first 3 days after *uncomplicated* major surgery in patients on an inadequate diet of 500–1200 nitrogen-free calories daily, are no greater than nitrogen deficits developing over the same period in age and sex-matched controls on the same diet who are not operated on. This suggests that the negative nitrogen balance in the *uncompli-cated*, early post-operative phase is due more to an inadequate diet than anything else. If these patients are provided with a minimum of 2500 calories and 12 g of nitrogen (72 g protein) daily, a negative nitrogen balance can usually be prevented.

The extent of negative nitrogen balance increases in patients with fever, major trauma, severe sepsis, or widespread burns, and these patients may rapidly waste, and die, from starvation. Nevertheless, even under these circumstances, adequate calories and nitrogen can very greatly reduce nitrogen loss, and here parenteral nutrition assumes perhaps its greatest importance. To maintain nitrogen balance in these conditions some 5000 calories, with 25 g nitrogen (150 g protein) may well be required daily.

There has been controversy about when to start intravenous feeding post-operatively, and clearly the loss of weight conse-quent upon 4 or 5 days of inadequate nutrition is perfectly well tolerated in the uncomplicated case. But, if it can be anticipated that the patient will be unable to feed by mouth after 4 or 5 days, then parenteral nutrition should probably be started immediately post-operatively. The expense is to some extent off-set by the shorter convalescence in hospital required by adequately fed compared with malnourished patients. When there is unexpected delay in oral feeding beyond this period, for

281

example because of prolonged ileus, or if at any stage serious complications arise, such as peritonitis, septicaemia or renal failure, parenteral feeding should be started. Otherwise accelerated protein breakdown, leading to cachexia, anorexia, hypoproteinaemia, oedema, anaemia and poor antibody formation, becomes a major factor in survival. Indeed, when more than about 30% of a normal body weight is lost, survival is exceptional.

Parenteral Nutrition in Inflammatory Lesions of the Bowel, and Malabsorption

Intravenous feeding may be required for example, in regional enteritis or ulcerative colitis when there has been severe weight loss, not only to cover surgical procedures, but also during acute exacerbations of the disease. In severe starvation, atrophy of the mucous membrane and muscular wall of the small gut occurs, probably due to their rapid protein turnover, and this must aggravate any existing absorption defect; but weight gain, and healing of previously indolent wounds, sinuses and fistulae may be achieved with parenteral feeding in patients with these disorders, even in the presence of prolonged ileus, sepsis and multiple surgical procedures. Parenteral nutrition extending over many months may however be necessary. But even over short periods adequate feeding can reverse a downward trend in regional enteritis, possibly by combating the effects of malnutrition on absorption from the small bowel.

Illustrative Case (HGH No. 022529). A 26-year old woman with regional enteritis was admitted to hospital in a moribund state, with severe weight loss, diarrhoea, vomiting and abdominal pain. Investigations: Hgb. 8·4 g/100 ml; total serum proteins 4·3 g/100 ml; serum albumin 2·1 g/100 ml; serum calcium 6·2 mg/100 ml; serum cholesterol 92 mg/100 ml; serum iron 66 μg/100 ml; serum folate 0·6 mμg/100 ml; prothrombin time 18 secs (control, 12 secs); faecal fat 18 g/day. She was able to take very little by mouth, and was given intensive parenteral nutrition for only one week. But at the end of this time her condition had improved and she could feed by mouth; after 8 weeks she had gained 7 kg, and thereafter continued gradually to regain her lost weight. The short period of parenteral nutrition appeared to have reversed the rapidly downhill course.

Parenteral Nutrition

Parenteral Nutrition in Renal Failure (see also Chapter 3). In acute renal failure severe malnutrition develops unless sufficient food is given, and, because of anorexia, vomiting and drowsiness it is often not possible to give enough by mouth.

The patient not requiring dialysis, but in whom urinary output is sufficient to allow an intake of 2 litres of fluid daily can often be fed adequately with intravenous hypertonic carbohydrate solutions and amino-acid solutions. The protein intake should be reduced to approximately 0·3 g/kg/day (20 g/day in a 70 kg adult) if the glomerular filtration rate is 5 ml/min or less, and the calorie intake should usually be at least 2000 per day. If urinary protein losses exceed 3 g/day additional protein equal to the loss will be required.

In acute oliguric renal failure the fluid intake must be restricted to a volume equal to the urinary output and other measured losses, plus 400 ml to cover insensible loss. Under these circumstances advantage may be taken of the high calorie content of the intravenous fat emulsions which can supply up to 2000 calories per litre.

With prolonged oliguric renal failure, or hypercatabolic renal failure peritoneal or haemodialysis is required; excess fluid can thus be removed, so the volume of intravenous fluid can be increased, but fluid balance demands close attention. Fat emulsions are again invaluable in providing calories. In hyper catabolic patients 30 g or more of urea may be produced daily, representing the breakdown of 90 g of protein, and with additional protein loss in the dialysate more than 100 g of protein may be required daily. The serum albumin gives an indication of the adequacy of protein intake. With haemodialysis it is important to remember that amino-acid and carbohydrate solutions are dialysable, and should therefore be used between rather than during dialyses. Fat emulsions can be used during dialysis as they are not dialysable, and do not interfere with the dialysing properties of the coils.

Parenteral Nutrition in Severe Burns

With severe burns it is frequently impossible to reverse a negative nitrogen balance even with a very high calorie intake until the

283

burn wound itself is closed. Nevertheless vigorous attempts should be made to do so as the continued calorie drain contributes to the demise of these patients. Severe base deficits are also likely to develop, and the more extensive the burn the greater the base deficit. This can be corrected using 8·4% sodium bicarbonate (containing 1 mEq bicarbonate/ml), and the bicarbonate requirement can be calculated from the equation of Mellemgaard and Astrup:

$$\text{mEq HCO}_3 \text{ required} = 0.3 \times \text{Body wt (kg)} \times \text{Base deficit (mEq/l)}$$

However, only about $\frac{1}{3}$ of the calculated requirement should usually be replaced.

Planning Parenteral Nutrition

Parenteral nutrition may be required over long periods, and therapy must be carefully planned to meet all of the body's requirements as far as possible. All the solutions used in parenteral feeding are in a water solvent so daily water requirement must be evaluated first. Most adults require 2—3 litres of water daily, plus water to cover any abnormal losses.

Accurate Fluid Balance Charts are Essential

Electrolyte depletion must also be made good, remembering that apparent deficits of sodium and chloride, judged on the basis of plasma concentrations may be spuriously high as these ions may be sequestered in intracellular fluid, bone and connective tissue. After severe injury most patients initially tend to be in positive sodium balance and negative potassium balance, and often have a metabolic acidosis. Electrolyte requirements vary enormously between patients, but generally 75—150 mEq of sodium and chloride are adequate daily, unless there are abnormal losses, for example from gastric suction, fistulae, diarrhoea or from the body surface. Some 60—80 mEq of potassium will usually be required in complete parenteral nutrition, even if there is no abnormal loss, as potassium returns to the cells with protein anabolism. (NB. 1 g KCl contains 13 mEq of potassium.) More than 500 mEq of potassium may sometimes be required to correct pre-existing deficits and to cover abnormal losses from the gut. Attention to potassium requirements is important as infused amino-acids are less well utilized when there is a potassium deficit. Magnesium deficiency is probably more common than is generally recognized, and 5—6 mEq may need to be added to each litre of infusion during the reparative phase after injury. After about a month of parenteral feeding trace elements, such as zinc, copper, cobalt, manganese and iodine, become deficient, and can be supplied by giving one bottle of fresh frozen plasma weekly.

Preparations for Parenteral Nutrition

1. CARBOHYDRATE

The commonly used carbohydrate sources of calories include glucose, fructose, alcohol and sorbitol. More recently another polyol, xylitol, has been studied but this is not marketed in the UK. Under normal conditions these are nearly equivalent sources of energy providing 4 calories per gram. Table II lists the preparations commercially available in the UK.

(a) *Glucose and Fructose.* Most adults can utilize 50 ml of 50% glucose per hour, and some can utilize twice this quantity,

TABLE II.
Carbohydrate Preparations Commercially Available in UK (1972)

	Cals/l	Cost/500 ml	Cost/100 cals
Glucose 5%	200	£0·20	£0·20
Aminosol 3·3% glucose 5%	300	£1·25	£0·83
Glucose 10%	400	£0·20	£0·10
Fructose 10%	400	£0·55	£0·28
Aminosol 3·3% fructose 15% ethanol 2·5%	875	£1·20	£0·28
Aminosol 3·3% glucose 15% ethanol 2·5%	875	£1·25	£0·29
Sorbitol 30%	1200	£1·00	£0·16

though glycosuria may occur for the first day or two. If 50% glucose is infused continuously at this rate it supplies 2400 cals/day, which is adequate in many patients requiring parenteral nutrition. There are many champions of 50% glucose, who prefer it to other calorie sources (particularly in the United States), but there are some minor arguments in favour of fructose. Fructose is said to cause less thrombophlebitis, possibly by penetrating endothelial cells more rapidly and thus exerting less osmotic effect upon them. Fructose is utilized in the absence of insulin, which may obviate the need for insulin when transient glucose intolerance develops, as after severe trauma and in renal failure. However, with reduced glucose tolerance there is usually an associated increase in the rate of glycogenolysis and gluconeogenesis, and thus a more rapid transformation of non-glucose hexoses into glucose. With frank insulin-dependent diabetes requiring insulin in any case there is no great advantage in fructose, and with ketosis most of the fructose is converted to glucose. Finally fructose does not produce hypoglycaemia after stopping the infusion, which may, rarely, occur after stopping a highly concentrated glucose infusion, because fructose does not stimulate insulin release. For this reason also utilization of fructose, unlike that of glucose is not impaired by previous severe malnutrition.

(b) *Sorbitol.* Sorbitol shares the possible advantages of fructose over glucose, being metabolized by sorbitol dehydrogenase in the liver, to fructose. Although sorbitol is not reabsorbed by the renal tubule its diuretic effect is small because it is very largely utilized when infused at rates normally used clinically (i.e. up to 500 ml/4 hours). Urinary losses usually amount to less than 10% of infused sorbitol. Clearly, if used in patients with portocaval shunts a much greater percentage will be lost in the urine, with a corresponding diuresis. In liver disease however, in spite of its metabolism in the liver, sorbitol appears to be well utilized, the activity of sorbitol dehydrogenase apparently being preserved, except terminally. Sorbitol may also be used in renal failure as there is no evidence of renal toxicity. It has been claimed that sorbitol causes less damage to vessels than glucose and fructose, and also that tolerance of sorbitol is not reduced during infusion of fat emulsions though glucose tolerance may be reduced. Sorbitol is conveniently prepared commercially in a 30% solution.

(c) *Alcohol.* Alcohol is a useful calorie source because of its relatively high calorie value (7·1 cals/g), and, like fructose and sorbitol it is utilized independently of insulin being converted to acetaldehyde, and thence to acetyl CoA. Alcohol is prepared commercially in combination with aminosol and fructose because it is oxidized more readily in the presence of carbohydrate. The concentration of alcohol is kept down to 2·5% because higher concentrations are irritating to veins. It has the possible advantage that it may make patients feel happier, but it is contraindicated in liver disease.

The various carbohydrate solutions should normally be infused at a rate of approximately 500 ml/4 hours. (Maximum rate — 500 ml/hour.)

2. FAT

Although intravenous nutrition using milk was first attempted in man by Hodder in 1873, in cases of cholera, further developments in fat infusions did not come until the 1920's, when fat emulsions were studied in Japan; in the 1950's they were developed further in the United States. Tables III and IV show the composition of fat emulsions commercially available today in the UK, and their costs. They consist of either soya bean oil (such as 'Intralipid'*), or cottonseed oil (such as 'Lipiphysan†), with an emulsifier for stabilization. Isotonicity is obtained by adding to the water phase glycerol, in Intralipid, or sorbitol, in Lipiphysan; being both isotonic and at a physiological pH they are less likely to cause thrombophlebitis than the hypertonic carbohydrate and amino-acid solutions. Synthetic triglycerides have been studied, but there is no clear evidence that they are superior to natural oils, and the current very high cost of producing pure synthetic triglycerides precludes their general use.

The original cottonseed oil emulsions had a number of side-effects which brought them into disrepute, though these were

*Vitrum, Stockholm.
†L'Equilibre Biologique, France.

TABLE III.
Fat Emulsions Commercially Available in UK (1972)

	LIPIPHYSAN		INTRALIPID	
	10%	15%	10%	20%
Cottonseed oil	100 g	150 g		
Purified soya lecithin	15 g	20 g		
Sorbitol	50 g	50 g		
DL-α-Tocopherol	0·5 g	0·5 g		
Soybean oil			100 g	200 g
Fractionated egg lecithin			12 g	12 g
Glycerol			25 g	25 g
Water to vol. of.	1000 ml	1000 ml	1000 ml	1000 ml

TABLE IV.

	Cals/l	Cost/500 ml	Cost/100 cals
Lipiphysan 10%	1240	£3·34	£0·55
Intralipid 10%	1100	£3·90	£0·70
Lipiphysan 15%	1780	£3·60	£0·41
Intralipid 20%	2000	£5·25	£0·52

largely due to impurities in the emulsifying agents, which have been eliminated from modern preparations. Today fat emulsions are of such improved quality that differences reported earlier in the survival rates of animals treated with the different emulsions no longer appear to exist. They are the best sources of concentrated calories, providing 9 calories per gram, and are therefore particularly suitable to meet high calorie demands, especially when fluid must be restricted.

Side-effects of fat emulsions, such as fever, nausea and vomiting occur in less than 1% of patients, and may be due to too rapid infusion — or perhaps even to the disease itself rather than the fat emulsion, being more common in patients with severe inflammatory disorders or malignancy. Although a slight, transient rise in SGOT and BSP has been reported in cirrhotics given fat emulsions, they very rarely affect a normal liver, and indeed liver function may be impaired more by starvation than fat, so that caution in using these emulsions in patients with mild liver disease may have been overemphasized. Nevertheless, in severe liver disease, and in nephrosis and diabetes, disturbances of fat transport dictate the need for caution. If fat transport is disturbed turbidity of the serum may persist after giving fat emulsions, and an increase in the α_2 lipoprotein fraction can be demonstrated by electrophoresis. Such turbidity may interfere with certain biochemical and haematological estimations, but these problems can usually be overcome by proper timing of blood sampling in relation to the infusion. In high dosage, fat emulsions may induce hypercoagulability initially, followed by hypocoagulability due to consumption of clotting factors. This is rarely a clinical problem because of the relatively small quantities used, but minor alterations in clotting factors may be seen, so that patients with known coagulation disorders should probably not receive fat emulsions. Deposition of pigment has been demonstrated in the livers of animals receiving multiple fat infusions. This appears to incite a microgranulomatous reaction, and such lesions have been observed in animals as long as 5 years afterwards. The significance of these observations in relation to humans receiving fat emulsions is not yet clear.

Fat emulsions are well utilized. They leave the blood stream rapidly, and do not accumulate in the tissues. Very little lipid is excreted, and there is a fall in the respiratory quotient and increased oxygen consumption associated with their use, together with favourable effects on nitrogen balance and body weight.

As much as 100 g of fat can be cleared from the circulation in an adult in 3 or 4 hours, and clearance is enhanced if heparin, which increases the activity of lipo-protein lipase, is given with the emulsion (1 unit of heparin/ml of fat emulsion). Doses as high as 12 g/kg/day have been used in fulminating ulcerative colitis, apparently without side-effects, but *it is generally recommended that the dose of a fat emulsion should not exceed 3 g/kg/day (or, approximately 1 litre of 20% Intralipid or 15% Lipiphysan per day in a 70 kg adult). The rate of infusion should usually be approximately 500 ml.in 4 hours in a 70 kg adult, and the maximum rate should not exceed 500 ml/2 hours. Electrolytes and drugs must not be added to the fat emulsions* as this

289

may break the suspension and cause flocculation. Electrolytes may be added to the carbohydrate and protein solutions, but care should always be exercised in adding drugs to the bottles, as some drugs may thus be inactivated, and if two or more different drugs are added to the same bottle one may inactivate the other.

PROTEIN

Some years ago carbohydrate solutions were used exclusively to provide calories in parenteral feeding. Then fat emulsions were developed, but it was not until later that we realized the importance of protein plus calories, in restoring nitrogen balance. Although nitrogen deficits can be reduced by replacing saline either with amino-acids, or with fat emulsions, a *positive* nitrogen balance will only be achieved when both calories and nitrogen are supplied. If insufficient calories are provided the amino-acids are utilized for energy and not for protein synthesis. Protein synthesis from amino-acids also varies with the body protein reserves, and although 50 calories may be sufficient to ensure the utilization of 1 g of nitrogen for protein synthesis when reserves are adequate, a much greater calorie intake is required in malnourished or hypercatabolic patients. Since patients requiring parenteral feeding generally fall into this category, *it is a useful working rule to ensure that 200 calories are provided for each gram of nitrogen.*

Protein, which provides 4 calories per gram, can be supplied parenterally either as hydrolysed amino-acids (such as 'Aminosol'*), or as a mixture of pure synthetic crystalline dl-amino-acids (such as 'Trophysan'†). Trophysan provides, in addition, carbohydrate calories in the form of sorbitol. Mixtures of pure crystalline l-amino-acids are now also available (such as Vamin* and Aminess‡) but they are currently very much more expensive. Some of the amino-acid preparations commercially available in the UK are shown in Table V.

There has been much controversy about whether protein hydrolysates or synthetic amino-acids are better utilized. It

*Vitrum, Sweden.
†L'Equilibre Biologique. France.
‡Astra Chemicals Ltd., England.

290

TABLE V.
Some Protein Solutions Commercially Available in UK (1972)

	Nitrogen g/litre	Carbo-hydrate g/litre	Cals/ litre	Na mEq/l	K mEq/l	Cost/ 500 ml
Aminosol-fructose ethanol	4·25	150	875	50	0·15	£1·20
Aminosol-glucose ethanol	4·25	150	875	50	0·15	£1·25
Aminosol glucose	4·25	50	300	50	0·15	£1·25
Trophysan 5*	6·48	50	364	6	8	£1·20
Trophysan 10*	6·48	100	564	6	8	£1·25
Aminosol 10%	12·75	—	330	160	0·5	£1·75
Trophysan Conc 10*	12·83	100	724	10	8	£1·57

*Figures for Nitrogen are those of the free α-amino nitrogen.

seemed likely that solutions of racemic mixtures of amino-acids might be relatively uneconomical, as the d-forms of amino-acids are poorly utilized. However, the d-forms of the amino-acids in the Trophysan preparations (excluding methionine and phenylalanine which are fully utilized in the dl-form) represent only about 10% of the total amino-acids, and part of these d-forms is utilized; also, a small proportion of the total nitrogen of a casein hydrolysate is in the form of low molecular weight peptides which are rapidly lost in the urine. *In well-controlled studies the differences in nitrogen balance using the two different sources of amino-acids are small,* and some of the reported differences may be due to other factors, such as differences in the nature of the illnesses, the degree and duration of depletion of protein reserves, the duration of nitrogen balance measurements, and the total calorie intake. If accompanied by sufficient calories both protein hydrolysates and synthetic amino-acids are very well utilized. *NB. 'Aminosol' contains 160 mEq Sodium/litre whereas 'Trophysan' contains practically none,* and added sodium is usually required with the latter. *There is virtually no potassium in either preparation.* Solutions of pure l-amino acids, seem to have a slightly greater protein-sparing effect than either hydrolysed proteins or racemic mixtures of amino-acids.

291

Side-effects from protein solutions are rare, but hyper-sensitivity reactions have been reported, which can usually be prevented by changing to another preparation. All these solutions are contraindicated in severe liver failure because of the risk of producing encephalopathy.

The quantity of protein required in parenteral feeding varies from 1·0—2·0 g protein/kg/day (70—140 g protein/day for a 70 kg adult, or approximately 1—2 litres 10% Aminosol or Trophysan Conc 10/day for a 70 kg adult), except in some cases of renal failure (see page 283). *The rate of infusion should not exceed 500 ml/4 hours.*

Occasionally it is necessary to give concentrated albumin (20%), not for nutritional purposes, but rapidly to increase plasma osmotic pressure. Albumin must undergo time and energy consuming conversion before it can be utilized for protein synthesis, but it may be useful to reverse severe hypo-proteinaemia, particularly in burns or ulcerative colitis, and thus prevent oedema formation.

4. VITAMINS

With long-term parenteral nutrition supplementary vitamins are needed. Ten ml of a preparation of the B and C vitamins, such as 'Parentrovite'* given twice weekly is usually adequate.

It may seem difficult with the variety of solutions available for parenteral nutrition, to know which to choose! Two suitable regimes for complete parenteral nutrition are shown in Table VI. Each has approximately the same calorie and nitrogen content, one employing a casein hydrolysate, a soya bean emulsion, and aminosol-fructose-ethanol — the other a solution of crystalline amino-acids, a cottonseed oil emulsion and sorbitol. These different constituents can of course be used in various other combinations, and the quantities increased to meet higher calorie demands, providing that 200 calories are supplied for each gram of nitrogen. Where such a high calorie intake is not required, the cost can be considerably reduced by cutting out the fat emulsions and increasing the carbohydrate calories.

*Vitamins Ltd., London.

TABLE VI.
Suggested Regimes for Parenteral Feeding

I	Vol (ml)	Carbo-hydrate (g)	Nitrogen (g)	Calories	Sodium (mEq/1)	Cost
Trophysan Conc 10	1000	100	12·83	724	10	£3·14
Lipiphysan 15%	500	—	—	890	—	£3·60
Sorbitol 30%	1000	150	—	1200	—	£2·00
	2500	250	12·83	2814	10	£8·74
II						
Aminosol-fructose ethanol	1500	225	6·375	1315	75	£3·60
Aminosol 10%	500	—	6·375	165	80	£1·75
Intralipid 20%	500	—	—	1000	—	£5·25
	2500	225	12·75	2480	155	£10·60

MANAGEMENT OF THE INFUSION

1. Veins are irritated by hypertonic solutions, producing thrombophlebitis. Always introduce the infusion directly into the superior vena cava via a wide-bore catheter.
2. Make sure that infusions are not run above the recommended rate.
3. Introduce the catheter with a strict, sterile technique.
4. Avoid lower extremity catheters whenever possible.
5. Keep the puncture site scrupulously clean.
6. In long-term feeding change the dressing over the puncture site, and the intravenous tubing every 3 days.
7. When changing the dressing clean the skin carefully with iodine and apply gentamicin ointment before covering with a sterile occlusive dressing.
8. Consider replacing the catheter in case of unexplained fever.
9. Do not withdraw blood samples from the catheter if it can be avoided.
10. Avoid contamination when adding medications to the solutions, or when injecting them through the tubing.

If these rules are observed veins can remain patent for months.
In conclusion, life-threatening complications may be a direct
result of malnutrition. The decision *not* to use parenteral
nutrition after about 6 hours in a patient who cannot be fed
otherwise — a decision to starve the patient — must be justified.
This does not of course mean that parenteral nutrition is justified in all such cases, and some of the indications have been
discussed. Parenteral feeding demands careful planning,
scrupulous technique, close supervision and frequent reappraisal
as the situation is not static. Properly used it can be life-saving.

FURTHER READING

Parenteral Nutrition (1970). *Proceedings of an International Symposium,*
    Vanderbilt University School of Medicine, Nashville, Tennessee.
    Ed. H. C. Meng & D. H. Law. Charles C. Thomas, Springfield, Illinois,
    USA.
Symposium on parenteral nutrition arranged by the Norwegian Gastro-
    enterological Society (1969). *Scand. J. Gastroent.,* **4.** (Suppl. 3).

Index

Index